FORGET THE FEAR OF FOOD

FORGET THE FEAR OF

FOOD

DR. CHRISTINE FENN

FRSH, FRGS

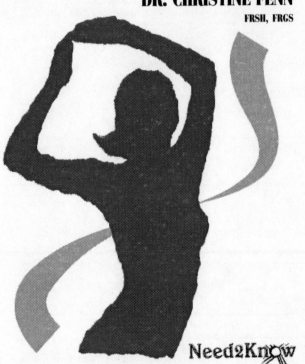

Need2Know

HARNESS THE POWER OF MIND AND BODY

© Dr Christine Fenn 1997

First published by Need2Know 1997
This edition published by Need2Know 1998
Need2Know, 1-2 Wainman Road, Woodston,
Peterborough PE2 7BU

Edited by Anne Sandys
Typesetting by Forward Press Ltd

Contents

To Mum and Dad for their love and support in everything I do.

To everyone who wants to stop dieting and start living!

Why walk when you can fly?

Author Acknowledgement

I am forever indebted and a millions thanks to my dear friend Jean Stewart for taking the time to read the raw manuscript and for her valuable comments.

Christine Fenn

Introduction

In today's modern society, there are two types of women; those who are watching their weight, and those who pretend not to be. For a long time now, we have also been told that there are basically two ways to lose weight. On one hand was the safe and effective method - which worked. It involved slow, steady weight loss and relied on continuous drudgery and self-denial - hardly the happiest time of your life! The other was the opposite. The quick fix of diet pills, milkshakes or some magic formula based on an extract of South American seaweed that promised to trim you effortlessly. Above all, it was so easy and so quick that you could get on with the rest of your life without even being aware that you were 'on a diet!'

This book is for those who have tried both methods . . . and failed. You may have lost weight, but you are still not happy with yourself. Something is wrong, missing or not quite right with your life but you can't put your finger on it. You will find out not only about food and dieting but also about yourself and how this affects what you eat.

Do you look in the mirror every day and say to yourself 'Wow, you look great. What a lovely face and such a fabulous figure'? If so, this book is *not* for you! Put it down immediately and get on with your life. If you already feel good about yourself, glowing with self-esteem and happy with your body, you won't be able to relate to any of these chapters at all. You cannot understand why the rest of us spend most of our adult lives worrying about the shape of our nose, eyes and mouth or the size of our hips, thighs, tummy and double chin.

Or . . .

do you look in a full length mirror and think,

'Oh no. I am so fat, I must go on a diet!'

Do other people give you genuine, heartfelt compliments, which you instantly refuse as you tell them 'the truth' about yourself pointing out all the bits that wobble, flab or rub together as irrefutable *evidence*?

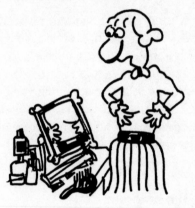

If you always *see* yourself in the worst possible light, whilst others say how wonderful you look, join the club - this book is for you.

Have you ever tried to lose weight before . . . and failed? No doubt you already have a hefty selection of diet books that promise 'the *easy* way to slim' or '*the latest* diet discovery - lose weight fast without hunger' . . . which for some reason have not kept that promise. The very fact that some diet plans have a sequel implies that the first one didn't work!

They may have left you feeling a failure, worthless and

with your self-esteem in tatters. This book is different. It concerns feeling good about yourself and getting your eating habits sorted out - for life. It is about taking the guilt out of eating and putting the enjoyment back in.

Have you ever wondered in exasperation why we put on weight in the first place?

'That's easy' you might say, 'we get fat because we eat too much.'

This is basically true, but go a little further and ask yourself *why* it is that we eat too much. How do we control our food intake? What makes us stop eating? Do we only eat when we are hungry? How can modern processed food encourage you to overeat and ultimately, why does dieting make you fat? This book will give you the answers. Part I deals with the problems - why we put on weight. Part II will give you the solutions.

Obesity - the big problem

There is no doubt that many people in the UK are overweight or obese, and that their health would benefit if they lost weight. For others, dieting has become a preoccupation, a way of life, an obsession - which creates more problems than it has the potential to solve. It is important to identify if you are overweight in your mind or on the bathroom scales. You need to examine what 'being fat' means to you. At 5' 4" a woman who weighs 13 stones is fat. But a woman who is 9 stones 5 pounds and wants to be 9 stones is also fat - in her own mind. And if that is where the problem lies, in the mind, then that is where the answers are to be found too.

For many people, diets just don't work because they are based on a quick fix solution which acts against human metabolism rather than along with it. Chapter 1 will explain the dangers of dieting and show why, in the long term, you lose £'s not lb's.

Fear of food

So many people, when on a diet, are frightened by food - are you? Do you spend your days planning what you are, and are not, going to eat for the next 24 hours? Do you become terrorised by the thought of being asked out to dinner whilst you are 'on a diet'? You are fighting against food every day, with the horror of finally giving in always looming over you. You were doing so well on your diet, but finally you cracked and a forbidden morsel crept past your lips. At first you are almost elated - oh the feeling of relief, that your diet is over and now you can eat anything you want to again. Pretty soon this is replaced with a sense of guilt mixed with weakness and failure. Familiar feelings, which come when you have broken yet another diet.

And yet, driven on by the pressure to be slim, we continue to diet. These pressures come from society, and from within. Emotion has an important influence on eating habits - are you an emotional eater? Instead of reaching for the latest slimming sensation, perhaps it is your own attitude to food that has to be changed. Part II will show you that there is another way of losing weight and feeling good about yourself. A way of overcoming a fear of food and boosting your self-esteem. It doesn't involve expensive protein powders, extract of seaweed or a potent cream that promises to melt away the flab. It involves a priceless ingredient, *you*.

Don't be disappointed, or feel apprehensive, about the fact that *you* can be the driving force behind the *new you*. Think about it. Vitaminised milkshakes and meal replacement biscuits are a cop out. A way of pushing the effort of losing weight onto something other than yourself. The bottom line is that *you* have the power to be whatever you want to be. Slimmer, fitter or simply content with the way you are now.

This book explains how to be the person you want to be. It will give you the principles of healthy eating, combined with techniques you can use to change your attitude to food. After all it is your belief systems that shape your behaviour. Your mind and the way you think is a powerful tool for changing your eating habits - for life. Society has already brainwashed you into thinking that unless you are a size 10, you might as well give up expecting anything great out of life. This book aims to undo the damage and show you how to develop a more positive image of yourself, releasing you from the fear of food. Food will no longer be the enemy.

The final chapters will explain how to lose weight - if that is what you want. How to lose weight effectively, not by a quick fix, but by learning new eating habits that become part of your way of life, instead of just a temporary diet.

Part One - The Problems

1 DIETING - THE INSIDE STORY

- Playing the losing game
- Promises, promises - the diet illusion
- Pressure to be slim - then and now
- The diet trap

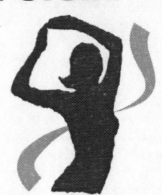

Playing The Losing Game

Dieters aim to be losers, but in fact they never win! The figures speak for themselves. There are more diets now than ever before and yet, as a nation, we are getting fatter! Statistics show that 90% of people put back most of the weight they lost within two years of starting their diet. This is because many of us do not know *how* to lose weight.

Starvation or fasting - the dieter's dilemma

The basic principle of losing weight is simple, you must eat less than you need. All diets therefore revolve around eating less. If a new diet is to catch on, it should have a gimmick, be effortless and above all, it must promise results . . . quickly. We live in a society where the pace of living is fast and we demand instant results. This is why the instant lottery scratch cards are so popular - no need to wait until Saturday. The great attraction is that you can find out if you have won *now*! In the same way, no-one wants to spend time losing weight.

If dieting to you means following the latest quick, miracle plan and severely limiting your food intake to strange combinations of food (such as grapefruit and boiled eggs; bananas and beetroot), you are on the road to nowhere. These diets do not work. You may lose weight initially but almost certainly this is due largely to a loss of water and, in the long term, muscle rather than fat. This is why it is easy to lose as much as 8 pounds in the first week of dieting. Muscle tissue is heavy because it contains a lot of water and glycogen - the body's carbohydrate store. Compared with our fat stores, the amount of glycogen deposited in our liver and muscles is very small - enough to provide about 600 Calories' worth of energy (men have more glycogen because they tend to have more muscle, and a larger liver, compared with women). Glycogen can be broken down relatively quickly to glucose, which represents an immediate source of energy for the body. If you severely restrict your food intake, your reserve of glycogen is used to provide energy, and the water stored with it is released. At the end of the week you have lost an encouraging amount of weight, but not much fat. This is because your body responds to a shortage of food in rather a strange way. Instead of burning up excess fat to provide the missing Calories, it is lean tissue, mainly muscle, which is broken down to provide energy. In this way the body sheds the parts which use up most energy - the metabolically active lean muscle.

Another response to starvation is to turn down the body's metabolic rate to keep energy expenditure down to a minimum. This is another logical adaptation by the body to a shortage of food. It is fine if you are marooned on a desert island and need to survive, but not so great if you are on a diet and live in the modern world surrounded by vast quantities of food. Have you ever seen anyone on hunger strike or a victim of famine rushing around with vitality? If your food intake is severely restricted, you feel tired and lethargic as your metabolic rate declines; you are firing on two cylinders rather than four. Unfortunately, the lean muscle tissue that is lost as a result of dieting tends not to be replaced. Consequently once you have reached your target weight and return to your previous eating habits, it is easy to pile on the weight - as fat. The end result is that you have changed your body composition. You have lost some muscle tissue and your metabolic rate never really returns to what it was before you went on a diet. What this means is that you now need less food than before. If you once kept a stable weight by eating around 2000 Calories per day, after severe dieting you now require only 1500 Calories.

The lazy way to diet

Most of the diets (Beverly Hills, Cambridge Diet, Slim Fast), involve a daily plan which tells us exactly what to eat. This, for the seasoned dieter who cannot trust themselves to choose food, is very reassuring. There is no risk of temptation because it is all done for you. You know that at 12.00 you will have a synthetic strawberry milkshake with a rather floury texture. At 6.00pm you will eat a diet bar with more Calories than a packet of custard cream biscuits and if you feel hungry in-between, just reach for the mineral water. These formula, slim-quick type diets sell in their millions but one of their many drawbacks is that they teach you nothing about healthy eating habits.

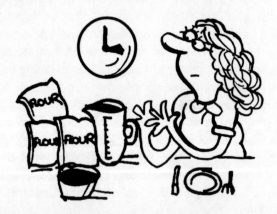

Once you have lost weight you can go back to what you were eating before which is probably why you put on weight in the first place. Since you need less food it is easy to overeat, in terms of what your body needs, and the excess Calories are deposited as fat. Yo-yo dieting means that you lose muscle and gain fat with every cycle of dieting. Just think how this affects your ego and self-image, let alone your body composition. A recent 4-year study lead by Dr Mike Green of the Institute of Food Research in Reading revealed that dieting caused mental pressure, stress and anxiety. The study concluded that dieters have a poor ability to concentrate; their reaction time and short-term memory are also impaired. For anyone who wants to get the most out of life this is hardly the way to live!

If you break yet another diet, do not expect any sympathy from the slimming food manufacturers. Their message is to keep trying . . . keep buying all the low-fat products, diet drinks and meal replacements. After all there is nothing wrong with the diet - it is just your willpower that is at fault.

Promises, Promises - The Diet Illusion

We all want to believe that there is a miracle cure, or a magic food, that allows us to eat as much as we want and still shed pounds. The promises that the new diets make are so tempting that we believe them - because we *want* to believe them. Every time a new diet book or weight loss system comes out we convince ourselves that this is the answer and religiously follow the rules. But whichever way it is packaged, the bottom line (no pun intended) is that dieting means deprivation.

For seasoned dieters, even the *thought* of going on a diet can put on a few pounds. The somewhat confusing headline 'Dieting makes you fat' is true to an extent.

Picture the scenario. It is Friday. Your clothes are tight and there is heaviness in every part of your body. You feel fat, miserable and finally announce . . . 'That's it, on Monday I'm going on a diet.' It's all systems go, but there are two days before then. Time to indulge. Knowing that after the weekend your life will revolve around cottage cheese, celery sticks and skimmed milk (all of which you hate), you stock up on a few pleasures before misery sets in. An extra cake, a few biscuits or that special helping of cream are acceptable in view of the impending siege to come. Already your mind knows too well the deprivation that awaits and has given you the OK to overeat. Even before Monday morning dawns you have put on a few extra pounds . . . even thinking about dieting makes you fat.

How can food have so much power over us? How can the same self-destructive diet-and-binge cycle continue? We deny, refuse, abstain, reject, weaken, fade, give in, eat, devour, binge, and suffer guilt and self-hatred. The apt description, 'yo-yo dieting' simply means that your weight and your self-image go up and down, but no actual progress is made. Magazines are full of stories of women who have lost 250 pounds - that's over 17 stones. It sounds impressive and you wonder how big they were to start with, until you realise that it is the same 50 pounds being lost over and over again. The sad part is that going on a diet and severely restricting your food intake means that, in the long term, you alter your body composition and lower your metabolic rate. With this type of semi-starvation approach, dieting really does make you fat.

Why then, if diets don't work, do we diet?

Pressure To Be Slim - Then And Now

Our attitude to fatness depends on our culture and where we live. In societies where traditionally food was scarce, being fatter than the average person in the tribe or village had several social and biological advantages - especially for women. The average adult female body typically contains a higher proportion of fat compared with that of a man. Pregnancy and lactation impose a huge energy drain on the mother and the extra fat that she had played a vital part in the survival of the foetus when the pregnant woman or her family ran out of food. Fatness in women is a sign and symbol of fertility, health and beauty. A large man is regarded as powerful, and as a result there are many rituals associated with feeding up an animal, a child, a bride-to-be, tribal chief or doctor. Our attitude to size in the Western world, where there is plenty of attractive and affordable food, is very different.

The abundant, throw-away era is over; it is politically correct to be green. To be conscious of the world's scarce resources and to limit your consumption of everything - including food. Magazines, newspapers and television carry images of the slim and perfectly proportioned. We are brainwashed to believe that slimness equals success. Think of Nicol and her Clio, the intriguing Gold Blend couple and the woman who dances lightly along the beach before tucking into a bowl of Special K. The message everywhere is that good looks and a slim body mean success and happiness. Above all, nothing wobbles.

Feminism tried to release women from the compulsion to diet, claiming that standards of beauty were dictated by men for their own sexual gratification and that women should be free to choose what they did or did not eat. But feminism is also part of the modern world. Theoretically, the glass ceiling has cracked, and both sexes should have equal opportunities at home, in the family and at work. Women can now have it all. However, the successful businesswoman is portrayed as tall, lean and above all, in control. Slimness, like the company car and expensive, well-tailored suits are hallmarks of success. Yet to achieve the right look involves a mammoth exercise in self-denial. Women are traditionally the carers, those who nurture and feed. They must buy, cook and serve food to their family or partner but they must not indulge themselves!

Mesmerized by so many images of slender, happy people we are conditioned to believe that this is the only way to be. Yet people come in all shapes and sizes.

Crows and canaries

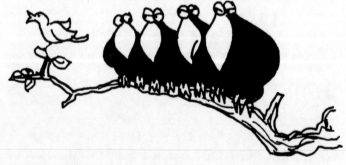

If you travel across the world there is evidence that traditional populations share certain characteristics. For example, Chinese women tend to be petite with a fine bone structure whilst African women have rounded buttocks and arms. The fingers and toes of Eskimos are short and thick to cut down the surface area for heat loss. This enables the Eskimos to work outside in the cold, using their fingers, without the need to wear clumsy mittens. Like it or not, you are born with a specific body type and shape that you cannot alter. Your genetic inheritance is therefore an important factor in determining your basic body shape and height. As one larger woman once commented, 'You can't breed crows and get a canary.'

The Diet Trap

Unfortunately a lot of self-conscious individuals repeatedly try to transform themselves into a shape that they just are not meant to be. This feeds the diet industry but ruins our self-image, and with each failure makes us feel even more inadequate. If you want to continue with this approach to dieting go ahead - it's a free country.

Rush out and buy the next diet book or tub of milkshake powder and push yourself through the agonies of deprivation, guilt, denial, and low self-esteem as you fail to maintain your (so-called) target weight - yet again. This approach to losing weight doesn't show you how to change your eating habits and how to uncover the reasons why you have put on weight in the first place.

2 FAT PEOPLE v THIN PEOPLE

- How big is the problem?
- What makes us fat?
- How much do you eat?
- Can we blame our genes?
- Your metabolism - fast or slow?
- Muscles - the forgotten movers

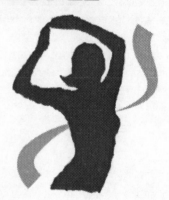

How Big Is The Problem?

The statistics show that we are, as a nation, getting fatter. In the 1980's 8% of women and 6% of men were not merely overweight, but obese. The recent report *Reversing The Increasing Problem Of Obesity In England* makes the disheartening prediction that, if we carry on in this way, 24% of British women will be obese in ten years' time along with around 18% of British men. Although there has been a boom in the health and fitness industry, it seems that we will be waddling into the 21st Century rather than leaping into it wearing stretch lycra leotards or track suits. Clearly, something has gone wrong and a change is long overdue. It seems that many of us have been trying to improve our eating habits - but not succeeding. Why is this?

What Makes Us Fat?

The simple answer is 'we eat too much' but this is not the whole story. How, for example can some people regulate their body weight to within a few ounces year after year, whilst others become obese? The answer is that humans are very well-adapted to conserving energy and preserving their fat stores when food is scarce. In today's modern society where food is plentiful, this may seem redundant but there are still many communities all over the world where village people are faced with famine and starvation if their staple crop fails.

Our fat cells

Humans are particularly good at storing fat. We have more fat cells (known as adipocytes), in proportion to our body weight, compared with animals that we traditionally regard as blubbery. Pigs, seals, bears and camels all have less fat, relative to their size, than we do. Only hedgehogs and whales have a greater proportion of fat in their bodies! In fact, it really doesn't take much for us humans to get fat. A single extra lump of sugar, above our actual energy needs, every day for thirty years would mean an increase in body weight of about 3 stones (20 kilograms). Putting on weight for some people can be a long, slow process. A few extra mouthfuls a day above your energy needs could result in a couple of extra kilograms at the end of the year. Put another way, to gain 10 pounds (4.5 kilograms) in a year you must eat only 50 Calories more each day than you personally need. This amount is barely measurable on a daily basis and yet over the long term can certainly mount up! On the other hand it is of course possible to pile on the pounds in a very short space of time. As we shall see in the next chapter, many factors determine what we eat, and how much. We do not simply eat when we are hungry and stop when we are full.

One man who was exceptionally good at eating (for whatever reason) and storing excess Calories as fat weighed 73 stones (465 kilograms). Not surprisingly he didn't get around very much, except for visits to the hospital where he was transported by fork lift truck. He held the unenviable record as being the fattest man in the world. This title is waiting to be claimed by somebody else, as he died in 1995. Even after his death, his size caused problems; part of his house had to be demolished to remove his body. He lived in America, a country well known for its larger than life attitude and a reputation for excess in everything - especially food.

Do fat people eat more?

All food is fattening, so why is it that some people (fashion aside) can wear the same clothes on their 47th birthday as they could on their 27th, while most of us associate more candles on the cake with more pounds on the bathroom scales? Many people claim they do not eat much and insist that it is their metabolism that makes them fat. Others maintain that they were born into a fat family, and blame their genes for their size. A great deal of scientific research has investigated the part metabolism and genetics play in the energy balance equation. Just as much effort has been directed to finding out exactly what, and how much, we eat.

How Much Do You Eat?

The classic way of measuring how much person eats is to
ask them to keep a food diary. This means writing down
all food and drink that is consumed over the study period,
varying from a few days to several weeks. Often the
'guinea pigs' taking part in the dietary survey are asked to
weigh everything as well, rather than estimating the
portion size of each food. Inaccurate terms such as 'large
portion of spaghetti' or 'medium bowl of cornflakes' can
mean wildly different things to different people! A
computer programme with a data base of the nutrient
composition of thousands of foods can be used to
calculate the number of Calories and amounts of fat,
protein and carbohydrate eaten each day. Measurements
of total activity and energy expenditure are also taken as a
means of crosschecking the results from the food diaries.

In people who stay the same weight for example, during
the study period energy intake and energy expenditure
should agree. In many cases they do not. This is
particularly common with obese people, who tend to
under-record their food intake by sometimes quite
incredible amounts. There are several reasons why this
may occur, but there is no way of knowing which one
applies. It may be that under-recording is due to a genuine
mistake, or perhaps a deliberate attempt to write down
what they think they should eat, rather than what they
actually do. Perhaps obese people are embarrassed at the
amount of food they consume and so adjust their food
record to cover up their true eating patterns? More likely
there is a subconscious barrier preventing them from

recognising their true food intake. In an attempt to overcome the problem of under-reporting, some studies have been carried out in a human nutrition centre designed as a small hotel. Volunteers stay at the centre where their exact food intake can be carefully monitored. The results from many (but not all) of the dietary surveys carried out in this way have shown that overweight people do not necessarily overeat, compared with thin people. These findings may seem surprising, and to contradict the commonly held belief that overweight do overeat. And they do not make the reasons for weight gain any clearer, as yet. What they do suggest is that the seemingly straightforward task of measuring food intake and interpreting the results is one of the most challenging faced by nutritionists and researchers.

Can We Blame Our Genes?

Recent cutting-edge research has concentrated on finding out how far our genetic inheritance can influence our tendency to put on weight. We have only 26 chromosomes, but thousands of genes. These are single units on the chromosomes and contain the coded messages that make us what we are - unique individuals. Each gene is special and is responsible for a specific trait or characteristic such as eye colour, height, body shape and now - the latest finding - a tendency to put on weight. Thanks to an important breakthrough in 1994, we are much closer to finding out exactly how much influence our parents have on the likely size of our fat stores.

A gene responsible for obesity in mice has been known for many years, but the latest finding of a similar code existing in humans has set scientists buzzing. Needless to say, the sensational discovery made headline news but it is important to remember that it is not a simple, straightforward case of:

- if you have the gene, you will become obese,

or

- if you haven't - you won't.

Identifying that a gene exists is just the first stage, the next is to investigate how it works. It could be that the gene controls a number of mechanisms affecting how much we eat. For example it may cause the manufacture of excess fat cells (which are then waiting to be filled), or affect appetite in some way. Those individuals with the gene may lack a chemical signal that tells them it's time to stop eating. By understanding how the 'fat' gene works, it would be possible to alter it and correct the obesity. Potentially, scientists could effectively use gene-manipulation techniques to enable obese people to lose weight permanently.

Even though gene therapy for weight control is still a long way off, it would not benefit everyone. Blaming obesity on your ancestry can only be justified for a very small proportion of the population - only a quarter of very obese individuals. If genetics were a major factor in causing obesity, then each generation would be becoming fatter. In fact, as a nation, we are getting fatter much faster than can be accounted for by genetics alone.

Your Metabolism - Fast Or Slow?

Talk to anyone who is overweight and they'll blame it on their metabolism. Metabolic rate is the speed at which your body can burn energy. Thin people claim that they have a high metabolic rate, whilst fat people declare that it takes longer for them to burn off Calories because they have a sluggish metabolism. To test this, Dr Andrew Prentice and his team at the Dunn Nutrition Centre in Cambridge set out to investigate if thin people really do have a fast metabolism burning off excess Calories as heat. Groups of both lean and overweight men volunteered for the study and were asked to live for seven months at the Nutrition Centre. During part of their stay, they were overfed by more than 50% of their own particular energy needs - that is one and a half times their normal requirement. If an individual needed 2500 Calories per day, he was asked to eat an extra 1250 Calories. The volunteers lived in metabolic chambers, known as whole-body calorimeters - essentially tightly sealed rooms big enough for a bed, washing facilities and an exercise bicycle. They had plenty of windows so that the subjects did not feel completely cut off and, of course, they could speak via a phone to anyone outside. They were under constant supervision, minute by minute, for 24 hours. They could not go anywhere and all their food was passed through a small hatch. This meant that the researchers could be absolutely sure of each volunteer's food intake. There was no sneaking out for an extra snack - or not eating the mountain of food that they agreed on for the purposes of the study. Not only was food intake measured, but all waste products and also the amount of energy used up throughout the day. In this study, as expected, the individuals who were overweight to start with gained weight. But so did the lean group! In spite of claiming that they could eat as much as they wanted, the lean men put on just as much weight as the fat ones (nearly one and a half stones in 42 days). Clearly, the experiment showed that the lean men did not have a fast metabolism which would burn off the excess Calories that they were eating. Perhaps the other side of the equation is true; that overweight people have a very slow, thrifty metabolism that makes sure any extra energy is efficiently stored in the fat cells? Again, volunteers agreed to live for several days in the special whole-body calorimeter chamber, and their metabolism was measured. Again, the results from these well organised studies are surprising. Far from having a slow metabolism, the overweight individuals had higher rates of metabolism compared with thin persons. This means that they also burn Calories at a faster rate compared with thin people. In fact overweight people need more Calories. They have more muscle tissue (which is metabolically active), and it takes more energy to move a heavier weight compared with a light one.

What is going on? It seems that the human body wants to be neither too thin, nor too fat, and has a remarkable ability to adjust its metabolic rate according to circumstances. This adjustment has also been found in people with severe illnesses such as cancer and AIDS. They lose weight very quickly because of their condition, but their metabolic rate is also lowered in an attempt to conserve their energy stores. In the same way, an overweight person needs to use up excess energy and so has a higher metabolic rate. When food is scarce, the body adapts to having less energy coming in by lowering its metabolic rate. The effect of this is to conserve the body's fat stores. As we saw in Chapter 1, this energy-sparing manoeuvre is the dieter's dilemma. You may be on a diet and wanting to lose weight, but your body does not know that. As far as it is concerned a reducing diet equals starvation, and it is unable to predict how long the starvation period will last. Its reaction is to adjust your metabolic rate and preserve its fat stores for as long as possible. This makes a lot of sense if you *are* starving. The ability to alter our metabolism according to the amount of food that we eat is probably the reason why populations throughout history have managed to survive food shortages and famine. However, with supermarkets, fast food restaurants and freezers full of food (all available 24 hours a day), the word 'famine' simply does not apply in most modern societies. On the contrary, there is the very real temptation to eat too much. An increasing number of people do, and consequently put on weight in spite of having a mechanism which turns up the metabolic rate to burn off some of the excess Calories. The research studies described show that our metabolism does its best to regulate body fat stores. Metabolic rate is turned down when we eat less (due to starvation or dieting) and is turned up when food is plentiful. And yet we still put on weight! Clearly there are other factors involved that must be considered. One thing that we know for sure is that we cannot take the easy way out and blame our fatness simply on our metabolism.

Muscles - The Forgotten Movers

Other research from the Dunn Nutrition Centre in Cambridge reveals that while our total food and fat intake has remained stable, we are much less active than we used to be. 'Britain slobs out' and 'Nation of Couch Potatoes' are common headlines used by the tabloid newspapers to describe the average lifestyle in the UK. We just are not as active in our everyday lives as our grandparents were. Our metabolism can cope with a large amount of exercise but it seems that we have forgotten how to use our muscles. We now watch an average of 30 hours of television a week compared with 13 hours in the 1960's. Newer and even more impressive computer programmes and virtual reality games are being designed. The trend is to spend hours in front of a monitor. This may challenge your brain but it certainly does not exercise your body. Central heating systems and washing machines have long since become the norm. When did you last chop wood or pound washing? Technology has taken natural effort out of life and we need to put it back.

The latest Government recommendation (published under the title *Active For Life*) urges us to build more exercise into our daily routines. Walking to work, a brisk jaunt with the dog, cycling for the Sunday papers can mean quite a significant increase in the level of activity for the average pomme de terre on a settee.

The 'take more exercise' is a familiar message. Those of us who have tried, tried and tried again to lose weight and yet cannot seem to shift those extra pounds already know the value of exercise in the energy balance equation.

Aerobics classes heave with bodies, the air thickens with sweat and the windows steam with the effort of Calories being burnt during a 40 minute work-out. Why then do we not shed pounds of flab?

Although we are responsible for what passes our lips (no one is force feeding us like rats in some bizarre, scientific experiment) it is clear that the type and the quality of the food is a factor in helping us to become overweight. Food used to be seasonal and wholesome, nowadays it is plentiful and processed. It is cheapened and adulterated by manufacturers anxious to maximise their profits, regardless of the effect of their food on our health. These products are available for us to take off the supermarket shelves and load onto our plates, or more likely eat straight out of a packet! The effects of these modern foods on our weight and our health are discussed in the next chapter.

3 MODERN LIVING & PROCESSED FOOD

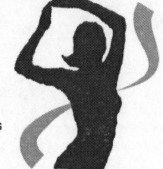

- The food we eat
- Starch
- Sugar
- Sugar and fat - the dangerous combination
- What's wrong with 'diet' foods
- Caffeine and the moody blues

The Food We Eat

Last year we spent £100 billion in supermarkets! Walk into a typical superstore and there will be 15-20,000 products neatly stacked on the shelves. If you are looking for a biscuit, there will be around 30 different varieties to chose from. Head for the breakfast cereals and there will be around fifty different types. Wander over to the butter section and it will appear to be shrinking as the tubs of margarines and the latest brands of low-fat spreads take over. Our food used to be eaten in the area where it was grown. The distance between soil and plate was a short one. Now we live in a complex world with complex food and distribution patterns to go with it.

Over the last half century one of the main changes that

has occurred is the way that food is packaged. Less and less of what we eat is in its original form, especially the carbohydrate in our diet. It is these changes that have had such dramatic effects on our health.

Starch

At the beginning of the century, we ate a lot of starch and it appeared on the plate as potatoes, porridge and wholemeal bread. Such foods are also good sources of dietary fibre, B vitamins and some protein. In the past, it was thought that starchy foods were fattening. Being on a diet meant avoiding carbohydrate-rich potatoes, rice, bread and pasta. We would take a large baked potato (which has only 150 Calories), and top it with cheese and butter or Thousand Island dressing (another 250 Calories). As we gained weight we would blame it on the potato. We now know that starchy carbohydrate foods are low in Calories and it is the amount of fat that we eat that makes it easy for us to put on weight. Fat in the diet is readily converted to fat in the body.

Another advantage of whole, unprocessed foods such as root vegetables, rice, beans, peas and lentils is that they contain 'slow release' starch. All types of starch consist of thousands of glucose units linked together into large, twisted chains. In this form, the molecules are too large to be absorbed in the intestine, which is why enzymes are needed to digest the starch. They break the links and release the small glucose units, which can then be absorbed into the bloodstream. As the name suggests, slow release starch is starch that takes time to be broken down by enzymes. This means that the glucose molecules pass gently into the bloodstream. This is how we absorb carbohydrate as nature intended. Thanks to the efforts of the food manufacturers, we are eating less and less slow release starch. It is extracted from cereals or potatoes, processed and distorted from its original form before being added to foods. This is wonderful for the manufacturers who use it as a thickener, or as the main ingredient in some products. This processed, cooked starch can be described as 'fast release' starch, which is rapidly digested and absorbed resulting in a sudden surge of glucose into the bloodstream. This is similar to what happens when a large amount of sugar is eaten - more about this later.

Maltodextrin is an example of 'fast release' starch. It is a pure, fine, white powder and behaves rather like wallpaper paste. Only a small amount of powder is needed to absorb an awful lot of water. Food manufacturers love it because, as most foods are sold by weight, this is a sneaky way of making large profits from selling H_2O!

Starch is added to so called 'healthy' foods such as fruit yogurt, cottage cheese, fresh soups and even baby foods! This starch is 'fast starch' because it is digested and absorbed rapidly, and plays havoc with your blood glucose, as will be explained later. From a nutritional point of view the added watery starch gel downgrades the food and literally dilutes the nutritional value. Maltodextrin is also slightly sticky which is the reason behind its other use - as gum on envelopes and postage stamps!

Sugar

Sugar is another ingredient which can be extracted from its original packaging (sugar beet or sugar cane), and added in huge quantities to foods.

There is no doubt that we love sweet foods - a newborn baby will suck vigorously on first exposure to a sugar solution. Humans have an inbuilt mechanism to prefer sweet foods. This is thought to be a hangover from when, as hunter gatherers, we scrabbled around and ate roots and berries. Taste was the mechanism to make sure that only safe foods were eaten. Since bitter foods were likely to be poisonous, these were avoided. Sweet foods were not only more appealing but more likely to be fit to eat. There are plenty of foods (honey, maple syrup, fruits, berries and dried fruits) which are naturally sweet. These used to be part of our natural food habits, contributing to the pleasure of eating by adding sweetness. The ingredients, in their original packaging, also provided other nutrients. Dried fruits are especially good sources of fibre, potassium and beta-carotene, which is converted by the body into vitamin A. Today mankind, especially children, loves sweet things, and the food manufacturers know it! They use enormous quantities of sugar, extracted from cane and beet to make new foods. These are known in the trade as 'value added' foods because they are based on sugar which is now a cheap ingredient. Undoubtedly our health would be better today if sugar had remained the scarce and expensive commodity it was when it was first discovered.

Ancient records throughout history speak of sugar as a honey running from a type of reed. It was highly prized and, in the Middle Ages, traders from all over Europe travelled to Cairo because the Nile delta was covered with sugar cane plantations. The crystallized juice became known as 'white salt' as compared with sea salt which was grey because it was unrefined. Nowadays the sugar on sale in the shops is made from either beet or cane. Tate and Lyle is the largest refiner of cane sugar and provides at least half of the sugar that is sold in the shops or to food manufacturers. Mauritius, a volcanic island in the Indian Ocean, is the largest exporter of sugar to the EC. The weather - hot wet summers and cool dry winters - is perfect for growing sugar cane and almost every field on the island has been turned over to growing the crop.

However, a strange thing is happening. Although less packet sugar is being sold, the average sugar intake per person has not changed. The average amount of sugar eaten is 40 kilograms every year, and most of this comes from the sugar added to processed foods. As fast as we try to heed the health messages, food manufacturers are tempting the next generation. Manufacturers know that children love sugar, and this is their route to introducing them to new foods. They also spend vast amounts of money to persuade us to keep guzzling familiar and unfamiliar sugary foods. It is not surprising that the health messages are being swamped by the powers of persuasion available to food manufacturers. Although the annual budget for health education is approximately £5 million, this is a mere drop in the ocean compared with some food advertising budgets. In 1995 Coca cola spent around £20 million to remind us that the 'real thing' was still available in its original glass bottle; £18 million was spent by

Beechams to launch their sugar-loaded Lucozade drink
into the sports drink market.

Sugar - pure, white and deadly?

Way back in the 1960's, sugar was accused of being
'pure, white and deadly.' There is no doubt about its
colour, but don't be fooled into believing that brown
sugars are any better for you. Most brown sugars are white
sugar with colouring added. It is true that unrefined cane
sugars, which still contain some molasses, provide some of
the B vitamins, and minerals such as calcium, iron and
magnesium. The amounts supplied vary according to
sugar type, with the dark muscovada supplying more, and
the light demerera less, for instance. But these nutrients
can be obtained from other foods which are a better
overall nutritional package. Sugar, whether white or
brown, refined or unrefined, is 99% sucrose, a simple
carbohydrate and one of the purest ingredients available.
It is basically a source of Calories. The claim that sugar is
'deadly' is a rather simplified one and needs some
explanation.

We have already seen that even tiny babies love sweetness
and many of us enjoy sugary foods. There is nothing
wrong with obtaining pleasure from eating, but the danger
with sugar is the very large quantities added to foods.
Sugar in itself is not deadly, but when used in such
excessive quantities, often in combination with fat, it
encourages an unhealthy and overwhelmingly fattening
pattern of eating. When food manufacturers add sugar to
their products they are adding pure Calories, often known
as 'empty Calories.' In effect they are diluting any other

nutrients also in the food. In general the more refined and processed a food is, the less nutrition it provides.

There are very few examples of natural foods which are concentrated sources of sugar. Honey is in fact the only one, but it is not naturally available in large amounts. Fructose is the main sugar in honey but is also known as fruit sugar. Fruit provides sweetness because of its sugar content, but the amount of sugar in a fresh fruit is small and is diluted by the water content. Fructose is slightly different to sucrose (the type extracted from sugar beet and cane, and found in the sugar bowl). Not all sugars have the same level of sweetness. Lactose, or milk sugar, is a very un-sweet sugar as it is designed as a first taste for young babies. Although we like the soothing taste, there is a limit to the amount of sugar we can eat before we find it cloying. If milk contained a very sweet sugar, newborn babies, who rely on milk as their very first food, would soon find it so sickly that they would stop drinking it. Nature has specifically designed milk with lactose to give a pleasant taste and to encourage the infant to take as much as it needs. Fructose, by comparison, is a very sweet sugar which means that little is needed to give a definite sweetness.

Most of the sugar we eat is sucrose. This is the sugar which is added to manufactured foods, or which we spoon into tea and coffee ourselves. As far as our digestive system is concerned refined, high-sugar foods are a new invention and one with which we were not designed to cope! Our metabolism in particular was not designed to deal with the level of sugar that is crammed into foods today.

Sugar blues

Glucose is the main energy source for the body. The brain in particular relies on a steady supply and cannot use anything else (except in extreme starvation). Because of this we have an impressive and sensitive system to regulate the level of glucose circulating in our blood. If the level of glucose rises above normal, this triggers the release of insulin, and glucose is taken out of the blood and stored in the liver and muscles as glycogen. If the glycogen stores are full, the liver is able to convert glycogen to fat - and we all know where that is stored! When the blood glucose level falls, another hormone, glucagon, is activated which causes glycogen to be broken down once again to glucose, which is then released into the bloodstream.

All forms of carbohydrate (sugars and starch) are ultimately broken down to individual glucose units which are absorbed into the blood. Not surprisingly, our blood glucose level will rise after a meal containing carbohydrate. However, the extent to which it rises will depend on the type and amount of carbohydrate that is eaten. Slow release starch (found in potatoes, wholemeal bread, beans, lentils and pasta) or fructose (particularly still in the fruit) is absorbed gradually. Blood glucose rises gently and insulin is able to make small adjustments to maintain a constant level. Highly processed foods, or those with a lot of added starch (such as maltodextrin) or sucrose, are very concentrated sources of easily assimilated carbohydrate and are rapidly digested and absorbed. A sudden, large rush of glucose enters the blood which in turn produces a surge of insulin in an effort to regulate blood glucose and bring it back to normal. However, the rapid release of insulin removes too much glucose from the bloodstream and the concentration falls too low. This is known as the 'sugar blues' or hypoglycaemia. The symptoms are feeling weak, faint, sweaty, dizzy, exhausted, anxious, moody, irritable and generally lacking in energy - and of course you are! The fast release, processed starch or sucrose that you ate has been rapidly removed from your blood, converted to glycogen and stored in your liver. The brain, being particularly sensitive to a lack of glucose, sends out signals to correct the situation. One effect of these signals is to make you eat something. It works - you believe that you need instant energy . . . and reach for another sugary snack. It is handled in exactly the same way as before, sending your blood glucose into a rollercoaster of highs and lows throughout the day. This pattern of eating can be very damaging in the long term, because of the erratic surges of insulin that are needed to control blood glucose. Today's 'grazing' habits, when the snack is a sugary one, also encourage poor nutrition. Eventually, muscles and liver become insensitive to insulin, no matter how much is produced. Blood glucose levels rise dangerously high and a condition known as hyperglycaemia results. Although plenty of glucose is circulating in your bloodstream, it cannot be used by the cells and tissues of your body unless insulin is effective. The insulin hormone works rather like a switch, controlling a series of gates on the surface of each cell, which can be opened to allow glucose to enter. The first signs of diabetes are an unquenchable thirst and the passing of abnormal amounts of urine, flooded with glucose which the body cannot make use of. The short-term damaging effects of eating sugary and highly processed starchy foods is that you are constantly reaching for more to restore your energy levels, as your blood sugar plummets below normal. The bottom line is that you are eating more than you need. Excess glucose is converted to glycogen; excess glycogen in turn is converted to fat.

Sugar And Fat - The Dangerous Combination

To add insult to injury, another thing to notice about many concentrated sugary foods is that they are also high-fat foods. It is this combination which is deadly because these foods are extremely palatable. They are very easy to eat - and very easy to overeat! Because they are concentrated foods, it is not difficult to swallow a great deal of sugar from a relatively small portion of food. Sugary foods are fast foods precisely because they do not take long to eat! A chocolate biscuit or an ice-cream takes only minutes to devour. Then having consumed it so quickly, it is not long before we are looking around for something else to eat . . . and then something else. Pretty soon, although we haven't eaten very much food in terms of quantity, because it was so very concentrated, we have eaten more than we needed yet again. One of the reasons why so many of us are overweight is not simply because of the amount of food that we eat, but because of the type. Modern processed food is concentrated food, no longer in its original form. Food in its natural state takes much longer to eat. For example, a 2-finger bar of KitKat takes about 20 seconds to eat and will provide 120 Calories. The amount of activity needed to burn this off is 15 minutes of moderately energetic step aerobics, or 20 minutes of brisk walking. No wonder people say that they do plenty of exercise but

Food	Minutes of exercise	
	Moderate level Aerobics	Brisk Walking
1 slice cheesecake	27	40
1 Cadbury's Cream Egg	28	41
1 cheese-filled croissant	31	47
1 jam-filled donut	26	39
2-finger KitKat	15	22
1 can Cola or fizzy drink	16	23
30g packet crisps	20	27
Small 50g chocolate bar	32	44
2 plain digestive biscuits	19	26
1 Danish pastry	47	63
2 Jaffa cake biscuits	9	12
2 scoops luxury ice-cream	37	49
1 standard size Mars bar	36	48
Bounty, 2 small bars	36	48
Bowl Frosties cereal	22	30
Bowl Coco Pops cereal	17	23
Bowl Crunchy Nut Cornflakes	22	30
2 Bourbon biscuits	16	21
1 individual fruit pie	51	68
McDonalds vanilla shake	44	58

The amount of exercise needed to burn off various high fat and or high sugar foods

somehow do not lose weight! They may be eating very little food, but if this is concentrated sugary/fatty food it is a never-ending battle to balance the energy equation and to spend around 30 minutes burning off a chocolate bar which has taken 30 seconds to consume. Check the table above for some more comparisons. The figures are averages, based on an individual weighing 68 kilograms

(10½ stones or 150 lbs). The exact amount will vary for each individual depending on age, sex, body weight and body composition.

Processed and high sugar/fat foods are concentrated foods. Change to eating real foods closer to their natural state and you can eat more food and feel more satisfied. The equivalent amount of energy in a 2-finger KitKat can be eaten as 2½ apples or 2 small slices of wholemeal bread, for instance.

And a small (50g) milk chocolate bar (265 Calories) is equivalent to:

- wholemeal fruit scone with scraping of butter and 1 teaspoon of jam or honey
- 4½ medium size bananas
- 6 large apples
- 5 nectarines
- 6 peaches
- 4 large oranges
- 5 whole cantaloup melons
- 39 prunes
- 20 toasted whole almonds plus 3 handfuls of raisins
- 1 large portion savoury stir fry rice with peppers, onion, garlic and tomatoes
- 1 large baked jacket potato with tuna fish or baked bean filling and a green salad (lemon and vinegar dressing)
- 1 large portion of fresh fruit salad with 1 carton (125g) natural yogurt or 2 teaspoons Greek yogurt

- 1 large portion of potato and courgette vegetable bake with oaty topping, 3 florettes of broccoli
- 1 large bowl of home-made or Baxters vegetable soup with a large crusty roll and scraping of butter

We live life at a hectic pace, few of us taking time to slow down and eat properly. We simply don't have the time to spend on preparing, let alone eating, a meal. There are plenty of foods on the supermarket shelves which are concentrated, pre-packed, ready to eat and require very little chewing and digestion. We are busy people, short of time, so thank goodness for all of these foods. If we choose sugary, fatty foods such as cakes, biscuits, savoury snacks, chocolate and ice-cream we can actually eat around 2000 Calories in less than 10 minutes. We rush around all day grabbing snacks and fast foods, whenever we have a minute, to keep us going. Chances are that we would have almost satisfied our daily Calorie requirement in the form of these snacks alone. Because of the speed at which we can gulp down Calories, it is easy to overeat in a short space of time! And yet, at the end of the day we feel justified in tucking into a lot more food because we haven't had 'a proper meal.'

What a crazy way to live. No wonder many of us find ourselves putting on weight.

What's Wrong With 'Diet' Foods?

Healthy eating is all about enjoying food and choosing quality ingredients rather than highly processed snacks. Making these changes can be quite a challenge, and a short cut is to fill your kitchen with diet foods, majoring on low-fat spread, fat free yogurt, one-Calorie cola drinks and crispbreads. What could be better?

The reality is that food manufacturers have yet again cashed in on our vulnerability and brainwashed us into thinking that these 'foods' are every dieter's dream. After all, here is a range of products guaranteed to take the guilt out of eating. We are seduced by the labels which proudly show that they are low in fat or sugar free. Unfortunately in the quest to avoid these Calorie-laden ingredients we have forgotten the meaning of good eating. Many of the low-fat alternatives to butter are foul concoctions of water and vegetable fat whipped and stabilised with a cocktail of emulsifiers along with plenty of preservatives, colourings, flavourings and added vitamins. Diet drinks are simply solutions of artificially sweetened and flavoured coloured water. How can these products, which are so heavily processed and so far removed from natural ingredients, be good for our health? They are not. And yet we are encouraged to eat them in the quest to lose weight.

Diet foods don't satisfy

The fact is that these low-fat and sugar free foods don't work because they take the pleasure out of eating. After a snack of reduced-fat cream of mushroom soup, crispbreads with a slice of half-fat cheddar cheese and a diet cola we are left wholly unsatisfied. Before long, we are reaching for a low-fat yogurt or 99% fat-free cream cake. Recent research has shown that far from helping a dieter on his/her quest to control Calorie intake, some diet foods actually stimulate appetite.

Other studies have shown that foods with artificial sweeteners were less satisfying compared with those with sugar. Guinea-pigs in a study were given a low-Calorie yogurt or one sweetened with sugar. They ate *more* food in the next meal after the low-Calorie yogurt to compensate and so at the end of the day, the total Calorie intake was the same.

Artificial sweeteners turning sour

They were heralded as the dieter's dream; sweetness without the Calories. Saccharin, discovered as long ago as 1878, was the first intense sweetener to be approved for use in food. Since then, other chemicals such as cyclamates, acesulphame-K and most recently aspartame (otherwise known as Nutrasweet or Canderel), have been tipped into our food. Nutrasweet is 180 times sweeter than sucrose (white sugar) and in 1993, 800 tonnes of it was added to foods in the UK alone. The desire for sweetness is big business, and worldwide sales of Nutrasweet have been put at $1000 million. Despite reassurance from the manufacturers that it does not cause health problems, there have been numerous reports associating aspartame with migraine, eye pain, headaches, and hyperactivity in children.

If you wanted to make aspartame you would need three

ingredients: phenylalanine, aspartic acid and methanol. All products containing aspartame carry a warning because 20,000 people suffer from PKU, a metabolic disorder, which means that they cannot tolerate the phenylalanine component. However, it seems that the methanol may be responsible for causing brain, eye and nerve problems. Methanol is a highly toxic alcohol (far more than ethanol which is the alcohol found in spirits, wine and beer). Methanol poisoning leads to symptoms of dizziness, forgetfulness, blurred vision and sickness. Other research has suggested that aspartame may promote brain tumours. All in all, a high price to pay for low-Calorie sweetness?

Caffeine And The Moody Blues

Do you wake up in the morning feeling sluggish and tired? If so help is at hand, and every day millions of people reach for the coffee jar knowing that the instant brew will give a kick-start to their day. This effect is due to caffeine, the world's most popular stimulant. It is in not only coffee, which provides around 100 milligrams of the drug per cup. A cup of tea contains between 40-80 milligrams, and cola drinks have around 65 milligrams per can.

The pick-me-up effect of caffeine works by raising the levels of two key stress hormones - adrenaline and cortisol. Modern-day living also keeps these hormones flooding through your bloodstream, and so caffeine is simply adding to stress. For some people the after-effects of a cup of coffee are not pleasant: feeling tired, grumpy, moody and irritable. Caffeine also affects the brain and so headaches, forgetfulness, and finding it difficult to concentrate are also common. Ironically these are the feelings which drive us to pour another cup of coffee or tea. Many dieters guzzle several cans of diet cola drinks each day, thinking that they are boosting their metabolism and controlling their Calorie intake. Caffeine does not stimulate the rate at which we burn up Calories; taking exercise is a much more effective way of doing this.

If you suffer from mood swings, headaches and lack of energy, it may be due to the effects of caffeine. The irony is that many diet drinks contain caffeine. One woman who wanted to lose weight became hooked on diet drinks. She was drinking 2 litres of diet cola each day and complained of feeling sluggish. 'I've lost the fizz that I used to have. I want to feel like a bottle of champagne rather than a soggy doughnut.' Once she gave up caffeine-containing drinks, she rejoiced at how good she felt ' . . . as though my system has been flushed out with spring water!' Simply cutting down on caffeine has produced noticeable differences, for many people, in their energy levels and being able to sleep better. But be warned, it is common to suffer from withdrawal symptoms at first. Giving up or cutting down on caffeine can make you feel worse before you feel better. This is due to the toxic caffeine being flushed from your system. But the benefits of feeling alive and refreshed by choosing caffeine-free herb or fruit teas are worth it.

4 HUNGER - NOT ALL IN THE MIND

- Why do we eat what we eat?
- Is there an appetite centre?
- Where does hunger come from?
- What makes us eat?
- Food wonderful food

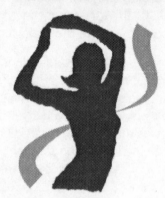

Why Do We Eat What We Eat?

Many people and normal rats (we know a lot more about rats!) are able to regulate their food intake and keep their weight within quite narrow limits. Rats are able to sense how much energy they have taken in and used up over a 24 hour period. If they are given water with glucose dissolved in it, they will eat less food to compensate for the extra Calories in their drinking water. This illustrates quite amazing control, and just how these small animals are able to regulate the amount of food they eat has puzzled scientists for years. Many experiments have been carried out in the hope that the results also apply to humans. In spite of all this research, we still do not know the exact mechanisms that make us start and stop eating.

Is There An Appetite Centre?

A popular theory amongst psychologists is that a small part of the brain is responsible for feeding (dubbed, logically, the appetite centre). Theory suggests that this area is active all the time and sends signals to encourage us to eat. The fact that we do not eat continuously, but have separated snacks or meals throughout the day, is because of the activity of another area of the brain, known as the satiety centre. When this is active, signals are sent which inhibit the action of the appetite centre. Satiety is otherwise known as fullness and is the term used to describe non-eating. The satiety or fullness centre is sensitive to signals from the rest of the body which reveal how full or how hungry we are. These signals include the changes in the levels of hormones and nutrients (such as glucose and fatty acids) in our blood that occur after we have eaten. Biting, chewing and swallowing also send signals - we often feel full and stop eating long before the nutrients from the food have been digested and absorbed into our bloodstream. Other signals, such as stomach fullness (there are stretch receptors lining the digestive system), also affect the appetite centre. It all sounds wonderfully simple, but the variety of signals coming from our bodies and pulsating through our brains are not the only ones that affect our eating patterns. What we think and believe about food is also a powerful influence. Although there may be internal signals which tell us when we are hungry or full, there are all sorts of equally powerful external cues that affect what we choose to eat.

Where Does Hunger Come From?

Eating is triggered by the way we feel and the purpose of eating is therefore to change the way we feel. Hunger is the sensation, the urge that drives us towards food and makes us start eating. At the most extreme stage is the wretched, desperate hunger state associated with severe starvation, in which we will eat anything. There are plenty of gruesome stories of individuals who, stranded and alone in a rain forest, will eat the maggots crawling from their open, infected wounds. Prisoners of war were certainly victims of starvation and there are accounts of the hostages chewing the leather of their boots in an effort to get nourishment. Happily, most of us have never experienced serious, prolonged starvation. Stop anyone in the street and they will find it hard to describe their own hunger, and yet claim that they are hungry. Others may experience a rumbling stomach or be aware of being somewhat peckish. These are usually only temporary sensations as, far from being short of food, we have a seemingly infinite variety and amount of food to choose from - and this can cause problems.

Supermarkets are stuffed with food - all year round. Delicacies once available only at certain times are now shipped in from all over the world in all seasons. New ways of packaging and preserving food make sure that there is plenty to choose from. If we want something different and really tasty, it is there for us to buy. With all this temptation and all this choice - what makes us eat what we do eat? If we can understand all the influences that affect our eating habits, we can begin to change them.

What Makes Us Eat?

Much of what we know about food is learned as we grow up. Unfortunately, some parents persuade their children to eat the healthy foods by offering a reward of a much 'nicer' food at the end of it! 'Eat up your vegetables, and then you can have . . .' puddings, ice-cream, sweets etc. We grow up to see certain foods as a bonus or compensation for eating the ones we don't like, or ones that we may *not* indulge in until the really nourishing foods essential for growth and health have been consumed. Pretty soon as adults, we can decide to indulge in the rewarding foods straight away, helped along by the power of advertising.

Eating with our eyes, ears, nose . . .

We are surrounded by sights, sounds, images and smells that constantly remind us of food. The thought of food, or perhaps just looking at your watch, is enough to make you reach for something to eat.

All good dieting books giving ten top tips to avoid eating put 'do not shop when you are hungry' near the top of the list. Walking around a supermarket, faced with all that food is enough to set your taste buds niggling for attention. Wander past the bakery section and the wonderful aroma of freshly baked bread is being pumped into the air to encourage you to buy. And it works! You find yourself reaching for a French baguette, warm and crispy, and you can't wait to get home and cover the soft, fluffy centre with butter. Other smells too encourage us to eat. Freshly ground and roasted coffee, the smell of toast or grilled bacon lingering in the air on a Sunday morning, all set your gastric juices flowing. Tempting smells, the sight of the packet of biscuits by the kettle, or the half-eaten bar of chocolate, remind us that food is all around us. The important thing is your response to them.

Food Wonderful Food

It was once suggested that the purpose of living is to avoid pain and seek pleasure. Eating certainly gives us pleasure. Depending on how much we like the food, positive signals are sent to the brain - and we keep eating. In time, most foods (no matter how wonderful) will finally lose their appeal, send a negative signal and we will stop eating *that particular food*. Eventually pleasure is replaced by monotony and we get bored with too much of a good thing. This happens with employees working in biscuit or crisp manufacturing factories. New arrivals on the staff think that they have died and gone to heaven when they are told that they can eat as much as they want whilst working. Most do, for the first day or two, but by the end of the week are sick of seeing so much of the same brand. However, not all foods have the same monotony value. Fat and sugar make a delectable blend and foods based on this combination can be eaten in amazingly large amounts - and on a regular basis!

Social eating

When the pleasure of eating is combined with an enjoyable social occasion, as it is when we dine out, the desire to prolong the event can encourage us to keep eating. If the restaurant is comfortable, the company amusing and/or romantic and the food well presented, it is not surprising that we opt for a pudding even though we may otherwise be well past our limit. However, in spite of a large meal, we may not necessarily have overeaten for the day. How many of us, knowing that we will be going out to take part in an event which majors heavily on eating, will curb our intake earlier in the day? This behaviour is related to another condition known as 'internal satiating', which can affect how much we eat. This has nothing to do with the food itself, but with what you believe about the food. If you think that a snack or a certain mixture of foods will fill you up, then it will.

We want what we can't have

Ask anyone who has been on a weight reducing diet what it was like, and the words 'deprivation', 'denial', 'forbidden' and 'restriction' come to mind. It is human nature to want what we can't have. When we decide which foods are out of bounds during the diet, we all know what effect this has. Somehow our mind focuses on the very foods which we have decided are strictly taboo. When we finally give in and allow ourselves to have them, we go overboard and usually eat far more than we would normally.

The sensation of hunger is not a simple one to explain. There are signals that come from within, produced after we have swallowed something, and sending messages to our brain. There are also all of the external sights, sounds and images that constantly remind us about food. On top of that, what we eat is affected by our own thoughts and feelings. In the next chapter we will consider another type of hunger that can also contribute to overeating. It is the hunger that is associated with our feelings and it is much more difficult to satisfy.

5 FEEDING YOUR EMOTIONAL HUNGER

- Food cravings
- Pre-menstrual syndrome and food cravings
- Stress and eating
- What's eating you?
- The binge cycle
- Eating disorders

In today's modern society, we are unlikely to be starving in the extreme sense, but people, especially women, are often hungry on a deeper level. We suffer from emotional hunger which concerns the needs of our heart and soul. Some people are hungry all the time - physically, emotionally and intellectually. They feel that their life is incomplete and, more importantly, they are not happy within themselves. To the outside world they may appear content, with a good job and plenty of friends, but their self-esteem is at starvation point. Not surprisingly, when people are this hungry they reach for food. They eat to satisfy their emotional hunger. They eat when they are lonely, bored, upset, angry, jealous, depressed, under stress or tired. But, unlike real hunger, no matter how much food you swallow the feelings don't seem to go away. We then experience something else . . . guilt! This is a wasted emotion. It drains our energy, saps our self-esteem and locks us into the downward spiral of compulsive eating, which is fuelled by negative emotions and the belief that another portion of ice-cream will be the solution.

Eating - and overeating - in an attempt to satisfy our emotional hunger is one of the main reasons why many people (women in particular) are putting on weight. Intellectual hunger can be satisfied, or at least fed by the consumption of books and knowledge from other sources, but where do we turn when we suffer from emotional hunger? Food is a convenient remedy - but only a temporary one. We need to identify the cause of some of these emotions and focus on aspects of our modern lifestyle that lead to emotional eating.

Food Cravings

Some people have a sweet tooth, others admit that it is much more than that - a fixation, a craving for certain foods.

Given a choice, sheep, horses, laying hens and cows deliberately choose one food over another. This is because they have a mechanism which detects which nutrients are missing, and they are able to select foods which will provide them. Laying hens have an enormous requirement for calcium, and they will crave any food which supplies it. Horses know that they must seek out the salt lick in the corner of the field in order to get the minerals they need. This phenomenon is known as 'specific appetite' and the closest equivalent in humans could be the food cravings that are so common during pregnancy.

The delights of pregnancy

The strange mixtures and combinations that an expectant woman would die for may be an indication that her body is lacking in certain nutrients. The powerful drive to eat a particular food may be a very effective mechanism to make sure that it is provided. However, although a craving for strawberries in winter may indicate a need for vitamin C, why is it that other foods which also provide the vitamin (kiwi fruit, oranges, blackcurrants), just won't do? It is also hard to see which nutrients strange mixtures such as banana and tuna fish pizza, often craved, aim to supply. This apparent internal nutrient sensitivity system does not seem to be activated only during pregnancy.

Following the birth of the baby, the mother suffers a rapid fall in the level of certain minerals and vitamins, in particular zinc and vitamin B_6. Low levels of this vitamin have been associated with post-natal depression. In an attempt to avoid the 'baby blues', or maybe because they are driven by a definite and quite natural craving, some women reach for a rather unusual source of the missing nutrients - the placenta! Some women swear by it and pack a large freezer bag before they leave for the maternity ward. Placenta cookery is certainly not for the fainthearted, or vegetarians. 'Take one placenta . . . ' is not the most appealing beginning to a recipe. When it is fried in olive oil, the taste is described as 'gamey' and a bit like liver. The ritual of eating the placenta is not a new phenomenon and makes a lot of nutritional sense, especially in developing countries where the standard of living is not very high. The placenta not only contains trace nutrients but is a rich source of protein, and is highly prized in some communities. Mothers who fear post-natal depression can turn to the old traditions rather than reach for Prozac; placenta eating is encouraged by the National Childbirth Trust.

Pleasure chemicals

The foods that non-pregnant individuals crave tend to contain a lot of sugar and fat (such as chocolate and ice-cream). This may be due to the particularly wonderful and sensual pleasure that we get whilst eating the food, but it could be more than this. Pleasure hormones, known as endorphins, are released when these foods are eaten. Opium is a plant extract and morphine a drug which work in a similar way to the endorphins produced naturally by the brain. They can help to control pain but are also thought to influence our mood and eating patterns. It may be that because the endorphins make us feel good, they then create a craving for foods which cause the brain to produce endorphins. Interestingly, anything which contains both sugar and fat is much more effective in creating endorphins than foods with sugar or fat alone.

Chocaholics

The ultimate pleasure food for a lot of people is the melt-in-the-mouth smoothness and taste of chocolate. It also has a unique 50:50 mixture of fat and sugar which produces a flood of endorphins through the brain in some people - no wonder they feel so good after eating it. Unfortunately, chocolate has an image problem: it gives you spots, can trigger migraines and makes you fat.

Things were very different 300 years ago. If you had gone to a doctor, you would probably have been prescribed a chocolate drink. This was because some of the earliest chocolate makers such as Terry and Fry were also apothecaries, and the sweet brown drink was given to help anything from poor digestion and sleep patterns to fertility and the delivery of babies. Further back in history we have Christopher Columbus to thank for bringing the cocoa bean to Europe. The chocolate he enjoyed was very different to the modern bars of Dairy Milk. The Aztecs drank it mixed with maize flour, chilli peppers and other spices. Later the flour and chillies were replaced with sugar and hot water.

These days we eat tons of the solid version. According to *Sweetfacts*, a report published by Nestlé, 46 KitKat bars are eaten every second in the UK and 6 million are produced every day to keep up with worldwide demand. For those people who admit to being addicted to chocolate, the nagging call of a Toblerone or Mars bar is as loud as a dripping tap. Why then do we love it so much? It can't just be that the stuff tastes so good. So does pizza and cheesecake but, unlike 'chocaholic', the word 'pizzaholic' is not officially listed in the English dictionary. Chocolate is one food that touches our soul like no other food can.

Studies carried out at the Brain and Cognition Sciences Research Centre at Middlesex University have shown that even the smell of chocolate (compared with other food odours such as coffee, baked beans and garlic) resulted in a reduction of theta brain waves, making the person calmer and more relaxed. Chocolate also contains several chemicals which have a powerful effect on mood. These include serotonin, caffeine, theobromine (which triggers migraine in some people), and phenylethylamine. This last raises blood pressure and heart rate but, more romantically, is the substance that is released when we fall in love! No wonder some people become addicted to the smell, the taste, the creaminess melting in the mouth and the feeling of euphoria that this luxury food brings. The confusing thing is that other foods, including dark chocolate, have higher amounts of these substances and yet it is milk chocolate that is most often craved. It may be the irresistible fat/sugar combination, along with the fact that we see chocolate as a forbidden fruit, that puts it top of the league of foods we crave.

Pre-Menstrual Syndrome And Food Cravings

Hormonal changes occurring throughout the monthly cycle could be why some women find that their eating habits go out of control and they start to crave foods such as white bread, ice-cream and especially chocolate. Certainly the hormones oestrogen and progesterone do have an effect on our food intake: they inhibit and encourage it respectively. As progesterone levels rise during the second half of the cycle, our appetite is stimulated. Our daily energy needs are also increased (by about 20%) at this time. Although we may need more energy, tiredness and fatigue are two symptoms of PMS, which affects millions of women between their teens and their 50's. Premenstrual syndrome is a collection physical and mental symptoms which can occur at any time after the mid-point of the menstrual cycle, and can last from a few days to as long as two weeks out of every month. Over 100 symptoms have been described including anxiety, depression, clumsiness, mood swings, bloating, sweating, headaches and food cravings. No-one is really sure what causes PMS, but there seems to be a definite link with nutrient imbalances. Women suffering from PMS were found to have lower levels of magnesium in their red blood cells compared with healthy non-sufferers. Magnesium is an essential mineral and is important in the body's energy production systems. It is also involved with nerve and muscle function and the action of some hormones. The best way to test whether magnesium has a role to play in PMS is to give magnesium supplements to women. It was found that there was some benefit, especially in relieving symptoms of depression and low energy. So it is not surprising that we want to eat food to put back these missing nutrients, but the puzzle is why sweet, sticky 'junk' foods and in particular, why chocolate? It is true that a bar of Cadbury's best does contain a reasonable amount of iron and magnesium, but the other highly processed foods have very low levels of minerals, compared with a large plate of steamed vegetables. Another effect of fluctuating hormones is a fluctuating blood sugar level. This may cause us to reach for the biscuit tin, but again other starchy foods (pasta, boiled potatoes, bread and rice) could also have the same effect. Somehow these foods just don't seem to have quite the same appeal! There could be a social explanation for high chocolate consumption amongst women just before a period. There is constant pressure on women today to be successful - at whatever they choose to do. Above all this means being slim and in control. While our friends, children, family, boyfriends, partners and husbands tuck into junk food, we remain in control. We restrict our eating, try to choose healthy foods and generally restrain ourselves from enjoying anything as wonderful as a bar of chocolate! But for a few days every month we dig in. This is the time when it is all right to indulge, because we can't help it. We can relax, pig out and not feel guilty. We now have an acceptable excuse - we can blame it on our hormones.

Stress And Eating

Stress is a wonderful thing. It gets us going, it motivates us into action, and sends our adrenaline pumping . . . but too much can wear us down. Stress itself does not affect our eating habits, but the variety of emotions that go with it do. Too little stress can lead to boredom and frustration - and the solution to these feelings is often thought to lie in the biscuit tin. Too much stress can mean being so busy and caught up in life's problems and anxieties that you only have time to reach for a custard cream between deadlines. Stress is the buzz word of the 90's - which is not surprising, considering the pressures from the society in which we live. Men are under pressure at work having to work the extra hours that used to be done by those now made redundant. The impossible task of doing more but to the same standards as previously creates stress, but also their role as earners is narrowly focused. They are programmed from an early age to define themselves in terms of their work. Often, they sacrifice themselves to gruelling work schedules and do not concern themselves with the everyday matters of running a home. Women have more choice; they can be workers and mothers with all the activities that go along with both. Monthly magazines are produced specifically for those who 'juggle their lives.' The image of the juggler is of a woman who calmly changes from her tailored business suit to sweatshirt and jeans, is able to change a fuse, redecorate the house, be a taxi service to Brownies, fund raise for the village hall and work out at the gym on weekends. Above all she keeps herself slim, fit, attractive and up to date with current affairs. She spends limited, but quality, time with her children and provides a listening ear and unquestioned support through all their teenage problems. She is, in short, a role model to which all women are expected to aspire. You can wake up now . . . or dream on. We all know that this doesn't happen in real life. Working women (high-powered or not) with families will tell you that they are permanently frazzled. They are torn between so many priorities that they feel they can never do anything properly. A day in the life of a flight controller at Heathrow is less frantic than that of a woman who must whizz around Safeway before a business meeting and then take a distraught child to the dentist. There may be some women who are successful jugglers, but certainly most are not. Having it all (at one time) is the female myth of the 90's, and eating habits are one of the areas to suffer in an attempt to live up to this myth.

Fast food is not necessarily junk food, but something which can be eaten perched on a desk, kitchen top or car seat and eaten in bursts whilst we do something else. In this way we can at least push food into ourselves whilst preparing a meal for the rest of the family, during work or on our way to taking parcels, pets or children to wherever they need to be. It is not surprising that we put on weight or find it hard to change our eating habits when we are not really aware of what we are eating in the first place. The only thing that we do know is that we are not eating 'properly'.

What's Eating You?

Reaching for food as a comfort has its origins in how we were fed as infants. When we cried, it was obvious that something was wrong, but our mother had no way of knowing exactly what it was. Maybe we were upset because we were too hot, too cold, in a room that was too noisy or we were simply thirsty. Whatever the cause, chances are that we were offered food to make things better. If we fall over and graze a knee, get cold and wet, or have 'been a good girl/boy' we are given something sweet or nice to eat as a comfort or reward. There is nothing wrong with this association, unless it gets out of hand. If we are constantly in need of comfort, we may be doing a lot of comfort eating. Food can also replace, satisfy and act as the nourishment in our lives that is normally provided by other people: love, affection, support, admiration, approval, friendship, encouragement.

The Binge Cycle

It is hard to define a 'binge'. To some people, it might mean a couple of extra slices of toast, whilst to others a binge can represent several thousand Calories' worth of food. In general, a binge is taken to imply eating a large amount of food in a short space of time. This is nothing new to us humans. Pre-historic man spent most of his time nibbling on roots and berries until an animal was killed. They didn't have the option of cutting it up and storing some away in the freezer for later. It was a case of 'hey guys, we just killed a mammoth - let's eat it!' Of course they then had periods of not eating, either because they were so full, or because there was no food available. This pattern of gorging and not eating is now repeated, by some of us, thousands of years later. However, the reasons for binge eating in modern society (where there is plenty of food available all the time) are much more complex, and relate to our emotional hunger much more than simple physical hunger.

Few people could claim that they have never 'binged' at least once in their life. In fact birthdays or Christmas are times when overeating is expected and positively encouraged. This is fine as long as it is part of relaxed enjoyment and the pleasure of eating and not associated with feeling guilty. The dark side to binging means eating a large amount of food uncontrollably in a short space of time. It has nothing to do with true hunger and, once a binge has started, it is difficult to stop. The 'mastermind' mentality - 'I've started, so I'll finish' - takes over.

Dieting and bingeing

Dieting and feeling deprived is the trigger for binging in some people, usually those who are preoccupied with food and are constantly worrying about their weight. These are the 'restrained eaters' who do not allow themselves certain foods and are in a constant state of semi-starvation. The effects of starvation are powerful, especially when it comes to food. What we cannot have (or do not allow ourselves), we want. This is the trigger to binge eat. It is almost as if the body knows that it has not had enough food and is trying to catch up - even if we are not hungry now. The extent to which people have problems with binge eating tends to reflect how they see themselves, their own self-image, and whether or not they are overweight. The real danger with binge eating is when it develops into the more serious condition of bulimia.

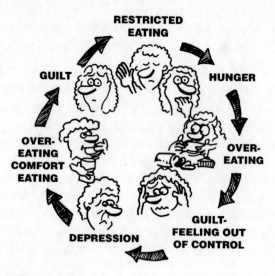

Eating Disorders

Ten years ago the terms anorexia, bulimia and binge eating disorder were hardly ever heard of outside the medical profession. Even for the sufferers, eating disorders were an intensely private affair. Each believed that they had some unique, terrifying form of madness. The good news is that all forms of eating disorders have come out of the closet. This means that they are recognised conditions and can be treated. A high proportion of sufferers do eventually conquer the illness, including well-known celebrities such as Elton John and Jet, one of the super-fit Gladiators.

One of the reasons why women could strongly identify with Princess Diana, and perhaps why they were so affected by her death, was because of her public confession of her eating disorder and fear of food.

The secrets of bulimia

Bulimia has some features in common with anorexia nervosa, although it is now recognised as a separate illness. Sufferers of both eating disorders have an overwhelming fear of being fat as well as an obsession with food. Bulimics are fixated by the contents of the fridge and regularly stuff themselves with vast quantities of food. They then get rid of the Calories, either by vomiting or taking laxatives. Neither method is effective as it is difficult to empty the stomach completely, and laxatives work in the large intestine. This is beyond the small intestine where most of the Calories and nutrients are absorbed. Getting rid of the food can cause a lot of physical damage, as a binge can last for up to 3 hours and involve taking in the Calories that others would consume in a week. One woman described what she would eat during a typical 2 hour binge: four or five Crunchie or Snickers bars, some Maltesers, a large packet of wine gums, a loaf of bread with butter or peanut butter, two large bowlfuls of cornflakes with milk and sugar. It is significant that many of the foods eaten during a binge are high carbohydrate foods. Some bulimics are physically addicted to their eating habits and claim that the food produces a definite 'high', although this does not last long and is replaced by feelings of guilt and disgust. One explanation is that binge eaters may have low levels of serotonin, a brain chemical which has a calming and soothing effect. Eating a massive amount of carbohydrate alters the balance of nutrients in the blood and leads to the production of serotonin. The binge may just be an extreme way of increasing the levels of this 'feel good' chemical. On the other hand, bulimia may also stem from the universal social pressures to be slim, from deep-seated anger, or a range of emotions that we are taught to suppress. Many therapists have had a great deal of success in treating bulimics through helping them explore any negative feelings of anger, low self-esteem or helplessness which they are unknowingly taking out on themselves through their bizarre eating habits.

Beating bulimia

It is estimated that 2% of the population suffer from this eating disorder, but over half of those who agree to have treatment recover fully. The first step in beating bulimia is to admit that you have a problem. Then it is possible to get help and break out of the trap. Sadly only two out of ten sufferers seek help. It is encouraging to know (according to Dr Fairburn, an international expert on eating disorders) that the majority of bulimia and binge eating disorder are treatable and the changes achieved are long lasting. He notes that one of the most satisfying aspects of helping people is seeing the person underneath emerge. Gradually the depression, tension and irritability fade, their concentration improves and they take a new interest in life.

Is dieting the sole cause of eating disorders?

Bulimia and any type of eating disorder may be a way of repressing feelings of anger, guilt and hopelessness, or a means to express those same feelings through abusing food. It has been said that Britain as a nation does not have feelings. Any population that can remain glued to 'Pride and Prejudice' week after week, or watch 'Eastenders' is certainly not out of touch with feelings. We may have them, but we turn to food to avoid the painful issues in life. This is not a new argument. In her book 'Fat Is A Feminist Issue' (affectionately known as FiFi, and first published in 1978), Susie Orbach repeatedly warned that we need to be in touch with our own emotions - and be able to express them. Orbach argues that for so long, women have been using their bodies to express emotions about their powerlessness. Even the most famous woman in the world, Princess Diana, admitted in *that* acclaimed television interview in 1995, that she did not know the words or how to deal with her post-natal depression and the lack of affection within her marriage. Instead she was driven to express these feelings through bulimia and self mutilation. As a result of regular meetings with Susie Orbach, Diana became free of bulimia and the cycle of self-hatred and punishment. Orbach helped put her back in touch with her feelings. Diana was able to show that, despite being a princess, she was normal. She did it simply by showing that she, like all of us, had emotions which she finally learned how to express.

Part Two - The Solutions

It is clear that, except for a small number of obese individuals, we cannot blame our metabolism or our genes for our increasing body size. Far from having a sluggish metabolism, fat people actually burn Calories at a higher rate compared with thin people. Experiments have also shown that when we purposely under-eat, our metabolism is very good at slowing down in order to conserve our fat stores. In today's modern society, this is not what we want. We follow low-Calorie diets in the hope that the less we eat, the quicker we will lose weight. If this were so, then the thousands of people who have tried this approach would be thin! Clearly the statistics for body weight show that they are not!

We now know that the crash diets of today closely mimic earlier times of famine, which the human body is designed to survive. Hoping to lose weight simply by trying to eat as little as possible is not the answer. We need to learn to express our emotions in ways that do not involve highly processed foods and we need to get back to eating - and enjoying - real food.

Our metabolism and the gene pool have not changed over the last ten years, but our lifestyle certainly has. The pace of living is ridiculously fast. Despite all the techno gadgets - computers, faxes, mobile phones and the Internet - modern living seems to need more than 24 hours in each day to get everything done. But we are human beings, not human doings. Many of our problems are the result of trying to keep pace with the incredible speed of change that is happening in society today. We race around at fever pitch and wonder why we have problems. On top of this we expect so much of ourselves. We want to be totally fulfilled and to be able to cope with everything that life throws at us. The reality is that we are only human and things rarely go to plan. No wonder we wander into the kitchen and reach for food for comfort and consolation. This, as we have read earlier, generates bucketfuls of guilt and disappointment in ourselves. So we resolve to 'get a grip', and mentally list all the foods we can and cannot have. As millions of people have proved, time and time again, this is the wrong approach. Using sheer willpower to deprive yourself of the foods that your emotional state craves will not work. Simply screwing your eyes closed and inwardly shouting 'no, no, no!' every time you find yourself moving towards the kitchen or nearest supermarket is not the solution. The conflict is between your left and right brain. The left side is concerned with logical thinking. This provides you with plenty of rational, sensible and intelligent reasons why you don't *need* to eat. The right brain deals with your emotional needs - never mind the sense of it all . . . this is how *I feel*. A real contest is on. Your rational mind says cottage cheese sandwich when, to your much more powerful emotional mind, only a bowl of ice-cream and strawberry cheesecake will do. Guess who wins? In this situation you cannot change by rational thought alone. If you could, you would have done it by now. You need to short-circuit the programme which drives you to eat when you are not hungry and replace it with a new programme that will provide you with alternatives. This means that when you are tired, take a break. When you are bored, do something else that is pleasurable apart from eating. Sounds simple, doesn't it? But it is not. Learning to address and answer your real needs is much more of a challenge than simply reaching for food as an anaesthetic. When you are lonely or fed up it is far easier to turn to a bar of chocolate than to reach out to others and perhaps face rejection. When you are angry with your partner, it may be easier to bury your head in the fridge or retreat with a jumbo packet or crisps. But these are only temporary solutions; unless you confront the underlying problem, it will not go away. A boring job will still be boring no matter how many cream cakes you eat. A bad relationship will not get any better if you make another doughnut the solution. The real issue is you and the realisation that you have the power to take control of your own life and how to want to live it.

Take the first steps to break free

It is time to develop a new enthusiasm for life and take a long hard look at who you really are. This can be a real challenge but if you want to break free from the grip that food has over you, to finally forget the fear of food, this is the way forward. It is not easy, nobody said it would be, but the results are worth it.

Elizabeth battled with food for years. 'As a teenager, I was chunky but loved sport and was happiest competing in all the school teams. I was outgoing, enthusiastic and popular. I had a passion for life and was born into the pile of human beings labelled 'achievers.' So no-one was surprised when I set up my own business, won major contracts and was invited to discuss topical issues on live television and radio programmes. I believed in myself . . . I had to. It was the height of the recession and while thousands of small businesses perished, mine did the opposite. I broke all the rules and became an accomplished career woman, with a wonderful family and supportive partner. To the outside world, I had it all . . . and yet I found myself turning to food. I became obsessed with eating and so scared of putting on weight. There was one rule that I couldn't break. The one in which society dictates that successful means thin. Every day, all day, I would think about food and work out how much I could eat without getting fat. Sometimes if I thought I had overeaten, I would try to throw up. That made me feel disgusting and yet so angry that food should have such control over me. I felt guilty and ashamed about my secret, and so could not bring myself to tell anyone. Life was a constant battle. I was fighting against eating and yet needing food to control my emotions. Modern society doesn't teach us to value our bodies. Instead we are conditioned to fight them and force them to be a certain shape, rather than work with them. One day, after 11 years of hiding and behaving 'properly', my best friend and I were talking about eating disorders. She then asked, 'So how long have you been troubled with food?' I burst into tears and babbled on about my binges and fears about food. She listened to it all and the relief of finally being able to tell someone was incredible. I think that just being able to admit to myself and then to tell someone that I had such a problem was a major breakthrough for me. I don't worry about my eating habits so much now. Every now and then, when I'm feeling low, I do still lose control over food. But at least I've admitted it to myself and I'm not so afraid. I call it my demon and can see him coming . . . it sure takes the sting out of his tail!'

Searching for demons

Where do our feelings come from? Where do they go? We don't often talk about our real feelings; it is safer that way. We talk around our feelings and either choose not to express them or don't get a chance to talk them through properly. Who has time to listen these days? We are all so busy trying to keep pace with the modern world. We are bursting with feelings - joy, pleasure, anger, frustration, hurt - but they have nowhere to go. There are some feelings (guilt, jealousy) that you don't want to admit to or talk about - so you turn to food. You soon learn that eating certain foods can change your mood and tranquillize your feelings. This is how we come to rely on food as a comfort. The reality is that our feelings haven't changed. What we have done is changed how we express our feelings. The problem when we use food to stifle our anger, resentment, depression, sadness, or loneliness is that it works - for a short while. But once you have stuffed yourself to bursting point, you are still emotionally hungry - plus you have the added feelings of disgust and guilt. Soon, food stops being a comfort and becomes the enemy. The food is now in charge of how you express feelings; you are no longer in control of food, it controls you. This is why dieting is the problem, not the solution. By focusing on what you can and cannot eat while on your diet, or using food as a medicine, you are avoiding the real issue - your feelings and how they affect you. *Simply being on a diet, doesn't make things any clearer, or help you face up to the real challenges in your life. All you are doing is adding eating problems to your underlying worries, which are not going to change.* You can kid yourself that whilst you are eating you feel better but, if you are really honest, you know it is only a short-term relief from your feelings.

So you have a choice. You can remain trapped, living your life as you do now and not making any changes *or* you can think about what you can do to change your life for the better. Remember, if you carry on doing what you have always done, you will always get what you have always got!

Ask yourself, are you happy? Do you look forward to work, enjoy a good social life, feel relaxed, energised and carefree? If the answer is 'not really' then something is not quite right, and maybe this is the reason why you turn to food, time and time again, and find it so difficult to lose weight. Simply by understanding how you are using food, and that dieting is not the answer, you have the key to making changes. Sometimes the simplest stories contain the lessons to be learned . . .

Here is Edward Bear, coming downstairs bump, bump, bump, on the back of his head, behind Christopher Robin. It is, as far as he knows, the only way of coming downstairs, but sometimes he feels that there really must be a better way - if only he could stop bumping for a minute and think of it.

Adapted from *Winnie The Pooh* by A A Milne

There is a better way and it means digging deep and being honest with yourself about why you eat what you eat. If you can uncover the reason(s) why you put on weight in the first place, this is the basis for changing your eating habits.

So, getting back to the original question, why do we put on weight? The answer for most people is a combination of:

- We need food to satisfy our emotional hunger. Is it our stressful lifestyle and suppressed feelings that drive us to eat what we eat?

- The type of food we eat.

The rest of the book will show you how to confront the reasons why you overeat and help you to make changes.

6 EXAMINE YOUR LIFESTYLE

- Stress
- Symptoms of stress
- Life's hard … and then you die
- Our daily stress

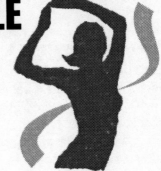

Stress

Out on the plains of Africa, prehistoric people must have lived in fear of their lives. With wild animals waiting around every tree or clump of grass, poised to pounce, you could argue that each day for these people was stressful! Not much has changed. Step out too soon these days and you risk getting run over by a bus. There are physical dangers, but these are rapidly being overtaken by modern-day mental threats such as fear of losing a job, of making a fool of ourselves, of not being a good enough wife, mother, partner, employee, friend or lover.

Certain jobs are dangerous or carry a huge responsibility, where a single slip or wrong decision can be disastrous. Individuals working offshore, air traffic controllers, long distance lorry drivers, doctors, policemen and policewomen carry burdens which can add up to enormous pressures.

The stress of change is another important characteristic of present-day life. Human beings dislike change and we find a new job, house, husband, or baby very stressful events.

What stresses us most?

Everything has the potential to make us stressed. Some people go out of their way to add it to their lives. Ask them, 'What did you do over the weekend?' and they might list bungee jumping, trampolining, parachuting, skiing, white-water rafting or mountain biking. Being an adrenaline junkie does not necessarily mean being active - just plonk yourself down in front of the nearest horror film. The fact that some people thrive on it means that it is not the stress itself that is the problem, but how we deal with it. Obviously we are all affected by stressful events such as a death in the family, divorce, or some sort of personal injury or disease. But certain so-called 'pleasant' events (Christmas and going on holiday) can represent major stress for some of us! The important thing is to be able to recognise the symptoms, identify what is causing them, and then do something about it.

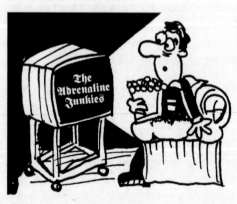

Symptoms Of Stress

Some of the conditions listed below might be due to other causes, but if you suffer from several of them at any one time, then stress is probably a major factor.

Physical signs

- Constant craving for food, especially when under pressure.
- Always relying on 'comfort' foods (chocolate, biscuits, cakes, sweets).
- Constantly gaining or losing weight.
- Indigestion or heartburn.
- Constipation or diarrhoea.
- Bloated stomach.
- Irritable bowel syndrome, IBS.
- Having trouble getting to sleep and also waking up during the night.
- Feeling nervous, fidgety and biting nails.
- Constantly feeling tired (even when sleeping well).
- Headaches.
- Feeling faint, or dizzy.
- Always getting whatever colds and flu are going around.

Mental signs

- Feeling anxious and trapped.
- Depression, crying or wanting to cry a lot.

- Finding it difficult to concentrate. Not finishing a task properly before rushing onto the next one.

- Feeling out of control.

- Being constantly irritated with other people.

- Not being able to relax, let go and laugh.

- Restlessness.

- Self-consciousness.

- Feeling ignored.

- Loss of interest in other people or other things.

- Feeling isolated and alone, even when with other people.

It is important to realise that many of these conditions are common in people with depression. There are several types of depression, including:

- Reactive depression. Triggered by a trauma such as an accident, a serious illness, a family break-up, divorce, or death.

- Post-natal depression. The steep rise and fall of female hormones during pregnancy can result in happiness in some women but depression (the baby blues) in others.

- Seasonal affective disorder (SAD). As the days get shorter around autumn, one person in 200 slides into this type of depression. It is linked with a rise in the hormone melatonin, a hormone which regulates our internal clock. Darkness triggers its production in the body and one effect of the hormone is to make us sleepy. In some people this has a greater effect and causes depression.

It is not surprising that when you are feeling low or under stress, you reach for sweet foods and comfort eating becomes a large part of your life. This could also mean that you put on weight - which only seems to add to your problems. The mistake that most people make at this stage is to go on a diet. They argue that at least if they lose weight, they won't look so bad and will have been able to achieve something. Wrong! In this state you *need* food. It is acting as a psychological crutch. Take it away and you are bound to fall. Your eating habits will sort themselves out later, your priority is to uncover the causes of your stress.

Life's Hard . . . And Then You Die

This is a rather negative attitude! As far as we know we only have one life to live, which is a good enough reason to take a more positive approach. Nevertheless, there are times when circumstances turn out to be more than just another of life's wet kippers that you can take in your stride. Major changes to your life do happen, sometimes out of the blue, and are a definite source of stress. Use the Life Journey Chart to map out the events that have happened in your life so far.

Overleaf is an example of a chart with significant episodes in life - some of which you may have experienced yourself? Now it is your turn. Use the blank chart to write down meaningful events that apply specifically to you.

It is easier to start where you are now and work backwards - but you can always add more as you remember them. Use a couple of key words to mark the

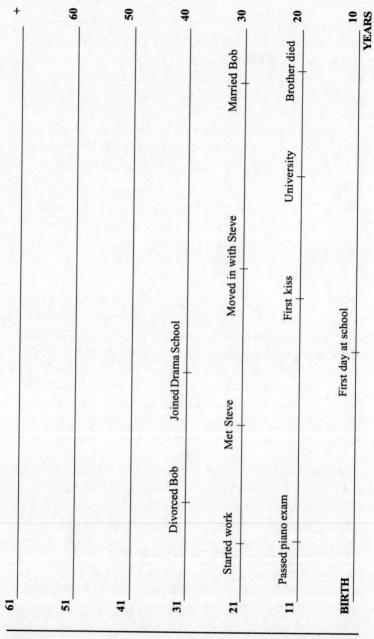

YEARS

BIRTH

10

20

30

40

50

60

+

11

21

31

41

51

61

occasion. Hopefully many of these will be significant and happy episodes (and will be a pleasant reminder of them), eg school prize in music competition, first kiss, passed driving test, fell in love, started my dream job, trip to Canada. The chart is useful to highlight events which may have happened to you recently and be contributing to your stress, for example:

- I left home or moved house.
- I got, or failed to get, a job I was going for.
- A close friend left work or moved away from the area.
- I had an accident.
- I was diagnosed as having a serious illness.
- I got married or divorced.
- An intimate relationship began or ended.
- A close friend or relative died.
- An important source of income was reduced or ended.
- I won ten million pounds in the National Lottery!

These are examples of events that can radically alter your view of life and/or your lifestyle. Chances are that your eating habits changed as well. Some people totally lose their appetite after a traumatic event. This is because whatever has happened (an accident, serious illness, losing your job or a death of a friend or member of your family) has totally taken over your life. You cannot think, or function as you did before. You may be able to carry on some sort of routine, but it is as though you are on automatic pilot. You are numb to the outside world and your eyes stare with a rather glazed expression. Your heartbeat rises above normal, you may become sweaty and then shivery, you become tense and your breathing becomes faster and shallower compared with normal. Your salivary glands don't function properly and your mouth becomes dry. Your digestive system shuts down and preparing or eating food is the last thing you find yourself thinking about. This is not surprising because your blood is primed with plenty of energy. The immediate effect of any sort of stress on the body is the well known 'flight or fight' reaction. This is the release of adrenaline from the adrenal glands (which sit just above your kidneys). One effect of adrenaline is to make the blood stickier which means that it will clot faster (it would have helped wound healing in our Stone Age ancestors). The adrenaline rush then produces a surge of glucose, released into the bloodstream, from the breakdown of glycogen stored in the liver and muscles. This is followed by a movement of fatty acids, which are released from our fat stores to provide more fuel for the body. All in all, the body is primed with energy and ready for action. However there is nothing for us to run from, or attack, to use up all this ready-made power. The best we can usually manage is pacing up and down, or thumping the pillow. This state of high anxiety means that adrenaline is constantly being released, and our bloodstream remains flooded with glucose and fatty acids. These chemicals stay in our system and we tend to lose weight along with our appetite.

Our Daily Stress

Hopefully, major traumatic events do not occur too often and generally we are faced with the simple, everyday pressures that affect us all. But if you are likely to react badly to stress, the effects can show themselves as moodiness, being irritable, feeling low, tense and generally 'wound up.' This is the time when your eating patterns can really take a tumble. You eat junk food, which makes you feel bad. You reach for something nice to make you feel good and you put on weight. You feel bad, you eat junk food . . . you think that if the world cannot be bothered with you, why should you be bothered with yourself? You need to break the cycle and firstly identify what is causing the stress. In other words, what is making you feel lousy?

	Event	Emotional Impact Score
1	My paid work load is excessive	
2	My work schedule creates problems	
3	I haven't enough time that I can call my own - 'me time'	
4	My outside relationships conflict with work	
5	I question the value of home life	
6	I question the value I get from work life	
7	My budget is too restrictive	
8	My friend(s) or family tend to rule my life	
9	I have ongoing problems with one or more of my work colleagues or neighbours	
10	I feel self conscious about myself (eg weight, appearance, social skills)	

Study the events listed opposite and consider how each relates to your situation. This is an opportunity to have a really good think about *you* and the way you live *your* life. Then give each an emotional impact score according to whether, or how, they have affected you in the last 12 months.

Give 1 for a low impact and up to 10 for a major impact. Only score those events that have occurred. For example, if your job demands more time than you want to give it and you feel that this is the cause of a lot of stress to you, then give a high score of 7 or 8. Ignore those items that did not occur, or do not apply to you.

The process of thinking about these areas of your life, not necessarily your absolute score, is valuable in helping you identify the possible sources of stress. We will examine later how your eating habits might be tied in with some of these. Nevertheless, your scores highlight areas of your life that may be contributing to excessive stress in your life. The simple answer is to make changes. Knowledge is power. Once you know what is causing the stress, you have the power to change things, although this is easier said than done!

Do you need a 26 hour day?

Many women are stressed because they are time pressured. Men are very good at focusing on one thing (usually their work or career). They leave the rest of life's trivia (shopping, cooking, laundry, filling the freezer, ironing) to somebody else. In contrast, women try to do it all, all at once. They weave their lives around their jobs, work, children, family, partners and social life. This leaves very little time for themselves. Time to slow down, to stop . . .

and relax. It is not everlasting youth or wrinkle cream that many women hunger for, but free time! If you have scored highly on numbers 1, 2, and 3 of your emotional impact list, then time management and lack of time is a major source of stress for you. Look back at the symptoms of stress, and if you suffer from tension headaches, feel constantly tired and find yourself eating fast, junk food because you don't have time to grab anything else . . . the answer is that you need to make time for yourself and learn how to relax. There are plenty of opportunities to de-stress and relax. There are lots that are cheap such as swimming or walking. If you can afford it, many new health farms and hotels are opening up to cater for the ever-increasing numbers of people who need to take time away from their stresses. There are a variety of walking and self-development holidays that offer a chance to get away from it all. They specialise in offering good accommodation in idyllic settings - such as remote parts of Scotland or the Greek islands - where you have time to recover and think about how to change the lifestyle that is causing the stress! A suggested list of these holidays is given in the Appendix.

In the meantime, go back to the list and underline those events that cause you stress and that you believe are in your power to change. Perhaps you have a lot of high scores, but not a great deal of underlining? Your ability to change things, to take control of your life comes from your own self-esteem and your own self-image. Building the confidence to make changes to the way you live your life is the first step, and will be discussed in Chapter 8. Once you can do this, changes to your eating habits will follow - and you may discover that you don't even have to resort to going on a 'diet!'

Fear

One of the most crushing emotions that we all have is fear. Everyone has been afraid at some point in their lives. It is that absolute terror that runs through your veins at the thought of going to the dentist or abseiling down a lighthouse. But there is another, more subtle, type of fear which many of us do not admit to but which niggles away at our soul and stops us from being all that we can be. What are *you* afraid of?

Check the list of some of the most common fears and, as honestly as you can, decide how many apply to you.

Fear of . . .

Being alone, becoming disabled, confined spaces, spiders, snakes, open spaces, success, failure, getting old, rejection, commitment, making a fool of myself, putting on weight.

Most fears are generated by our conditioning. All well-meaning parents urge their children to 'be careful' and not to take any risks in the big wide world. However, knowing where your fears come from is not important. What does matter is how the fear affects you. Fear is what tends to hold you back. It is as though you are well and truly stuck, knee deep in a large bucket of wallpaper paste! This gives you time to think about what you are afraid of and a little voice inside your head reminds you of all your nagging worries and 'what if's'.

Do these sound familiar?

What if she leaves me then what will I do? What if I lose my job, how will I pay the bills? What if I spend all my savings on a holiday? My friends will think I'm crazy. What if I go back to college and study for those exams? I'm sure everyone will think I'm mad. What if I accept a new job that takes me abroad, and it doesn't work out? What if I ask my neighbour to turn down his music? He won't like me after that. What if I go skiing and I break a leg? What if I tell him that I don't want to live with him anymore. . ?

Before long these thoughts begin to dominate your thinking. They serve to very effectively reinforce your fears and stop you from doing anything.

You are stuck, and find yourself feeling angry, frustrated and confused. Here are those feelings again; the ones we are not very good at expressing. Instead you turn to food as a remedy for your fears and medicate them by eating. So fear leads to anger, which takes us into the kitchen or supermarket to stock up on food to numb these emotions. This is how fear can lead to poor eating habits, overeating and putting on weight.

When you are afraid, you are out of control. You turn to food because it is the only thing that you think you have control of. Before long it begins to control you. It is time to face your fears and express your emotions in ways that do not involve food.

Facing fear

As Susan Jeffers explains in her book *Feel the Fear And*

Do It Anyway, fear is something that never goes away. This may seem surprising but being afraid is part of our growth and development as an individual. Although we cannot get rid of fear, what we can do first of all is to acknowledge it. The next step is to deal with the fear. Jeffers explains that no matter what we are afraid of, our biggest fear which links them all together, is the fear that we can't handle it. Turning this around - if you knew you could handle anything that life threw at you, what would there be to fear? This is the key to dealing with fear. Every time you start to worry and those nagging 'what if' thoughts jangle through your mind, simply utter these three simple words . . . 'I'll handle it!'

This is an incredibly powerful statement. If you say it often enough, you will begin to believe it and then you will really be in control of your life.

So, if you have a fear of food, a fear of putting on weight or fear that an eating disorder that you thought you had overcome might occur again, just remember the phrase, 'I'll handle it.' And you can. We can learn to face our fears and also express the feelings of anger and frustration that can arise from them. Up until now, you have probably raided the biscuit tin whenever you have felt frustrated, bored or confused. It is important that you acknowledge this. Emotional eating has become a habit for you. You associate a particular emotion (loneliness, tiredness, frustration etc) with food. The good news is that habits can be broken . . . once you know how!

The next chapter explains how to identify the emotions which trigger overeating for you.

7 THINK THIN

- Self-esteem - the key
- Take control of your life
- Ideal weight

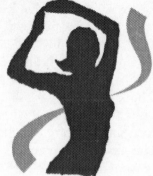

Self-Esteem - The Key

An important aspect of successful slimming (and the key to coping with eating disorders) is to feel good about yourself. Never mind what other people think of you, it is how *you* feel about *yourself* that counts.

Other people may tell you how wonderful you are, but you never seem to believe them! Admiring a person's good points is rather like handing them a present. It is considered very rude to refuse and throw their gift back, and yet we do it all the time with compliments! We also keep correcting them, pointing out our so-called weaknesses and imperfections. In time they may even begin to believe us, but what is more important is the damage that all this negative talk is doing within.

It is well known that how you think has a very powerful effect on how you feel, and how you behave. By constantly putting yourself down, you become depressed with all your negative thoughts and your internal voice drags you down even more. As you struggle with your weight or eating problem, those destructive thoughts then become excuses for putting things off and not living life to the full. This is the point at which you become a member of the 'if only' club.

If only I were slim, then I would . . . go out and do things, have more friends, enjoy going shopping, be happier . . . and so on.

This way of thinking only traps you into a vicious circle of waiting until you have lost weight before you can do all the things you want to, but you cannot lose weight because you are so depressed! Moody and glum are two words that would not apply to Victoria Wood. She is best friends with Dawn French, another woman who believes that good things come in large packages. Both are very successful and very popular comediennes, and Victoria has certainly overcome the agonies about her weight that used to bother her in the past. 'The worst thing about fat people is that they put everything on hold until some day when they might be thin. Meanwhile life is ticking along and you go on diets or whatever and nothing is happening. You think, one day I'll be thin and wear a bikini. You might just as well wear a bikini now.'

Self-acceptance now!

The way to break out is to change the way you think about yourself and build your self-esteem. If you do have a lot of weight to lose, it can be difficult to like yourself as you are now. However, the point is that you must try to accept (and like) yourself now . . . today. After all, it is *this* body, the one you are in right now, that is going to change. So you need to begin by seeing yourself in a positive light and knowing that things will get even better.

A good way to test how negative or positive you are is to examine your feelings vocabulary. Think about words you would use to describe yourself, using the list below. Aim to change any chosen from the left-hand column to ones from the right.

Feelings Vocabulary	
Negative	Positive
Pessimistic	Happy
Scared	Carefree
Vulnerable	Secure
Miserable	Delighted
Lost	Confident
Resentful	Trusting
Suspicious	Enthusiastic
Gloomy	Contented
Helpless	Powerful
Depressed	Determined
Apprehensive	Impulsive
Cautious	Elated
Exasperated	Fulfilled
Bored	Lively
Envious	Extravagant
Irritated	Pleased
Furious	Fabulous
Problematical	Adventurous

It is not only what you say, but how you say it. This adds
to your overall image, which also relies on:

- Your posture - do you slouch . . . or stand tall?

- Your expression - do you smile . . . or look grim?

- Your mannerisms - are you relaxed . . . or do you fidget?

All of these can signal a lot about you to others. Anyone
can buy the right clothes, but do you wear them with style
and confidence? It is often said that if you dress well, you
notice the clothes, if you dress with confidence you notice
the woman! Confidence comes from within, which gets
right back to the way you see yourself and how you think.
That niggling voice inside you (sometimes called your 'self
talk') can affect you in one of two ways; it can drag you
down, or be the source of your inner power. The words
you use in your self talk are a powerful tool that can help
build your self-esteem. This is because the capability and
potential of the human brain is awesome. Why not use it
to reclaim your image and develop a personal style that
suits you?

Working at it

There have been plenty of excellent books written about
the power of positive thinking. Many include inspiring
accounts by individuals who have changed their lives by
deciding what they want and developing a positive
attitude. If it is so simple you may ask why are we all not
successful, slim, powerful, rich . . . or whatever we want to
be? The answer is that one or two positive words now and
then are not enough. You must practise and use the words

and phrases regularly, so that they become part of your everyday way of speaking, reinforcing a positive way of thinking. Make it part of your daily routine, so that your new way of thinking becomes as automatic as having a shower, brushing your teeth or putting on make-up.

Maybe just now you are still a blob of negativity, doubting how on earth just changing your thoughts can change the way you live so dramatically. Think positively! You will be amazed at how it works! There are several ways in which you can weave positive thinking into your daily life:

- Listen to inspirational tapes. These are available from an increasing number of health food shops and via mail order. Listen to them in your car, just before you get out of bed or as you fall asleep at night.

- Read books on positive thinking. Some suggested titles are listed in the Appendix.

- Adopt your own positive quotes and affirmations.

Positive quotes

Words, in the form of poems, stories or single sentences touch us in different ways. Find some positive quotes that inspire you personally. For example,

'I can because I think I can.'

'I can complain because rose bushes have thorns . . . or rejoice because the thornbush has a rose . . . it is all up to me.'

'You cannot discover new oceans unless you have the courage to lose sight of the shore.'

'The key to happiness is having dreams . . . the key to success is making dreams come true.'

'You are becoming successful the minute you start moving toward a worthwhile goal.'

'Success is the journey, not the destination.'

Affirmations

Affirmations are also useful because they are statements of your own self talk. They are sayings that describe what is happening to you right now. They do not refer to what has happened in the past or set out what will occur in the future; they are positive statements that something is already happening. It is up to you to think up your own affirmations, but they may include things like:

- I am feeling fit and healthy
- I feel strong and in control
- I am becoming more confident every day
- I feel wonderful!

Remember - whatever your affirmations, they must be positive and relate to the present. Obviously you can change them as your situation changes, and to fit in with whatever feels right at the time. The best time to use or repeat these affirmations to yourself is first thing in the morning, as part of your normal routine. This helps to put you in a positive frame of mind and beats thinking 'lousy' thoughts. Another valuable way of strengthening your affirmations is via your imagination. Visualising and forming an image in your mind as to how you would like to be makes the affirmations even more powerful. It is helpful if you can close your eyes for this, and it is something that you can do whilst travelling in a bus or train.

For example, if you affirm, 'I am feeling fit and healthy' then imagine yourself exactly like that. See yourself fit and healthy. Visualise the clothes you are wearing and how good you look in them. Notice how healthy your hair is, the glow of your skin, and the sparkle in your eyes. Feel the health and the strength in your body, and notice how you stand tall and confident in the body of the *new you*. Now repeat this visualisation, but this time make the image of yourself even bigger - make it life-size. As you practice this technique, make the image of yourself bigger, better and brighter each time. This will increase the power of the visualisation and send messages to your brain of how you would like to be. The more you use the tapes, read books, use affirmations and visualisations, the sooner you will begin to notice a real improvement.

Take Control Of Your Life

Once you begin to like yourself, you become more self-assured. This puts you in control, and a self-assured woman who is in control of her life draws other people like a magnet! Now things are beginning to change and you can cancel your membership of the 'if only' club. Chances are that you may be the same weight as you were before but you have begun to lose the negative attitude to yourself. You feel good inside, which shows on the outside - and you can believe the very real compliments that you are getting.

Talk first, act later

Notice that we have not mentioned anything about what to eat (or what not to eat) during this period of positive thinking. This is because, by changing the way you see yourself, you can literally talk yourself out of feeling low, bored, tired, worthless, or lonely. These were probably some of the reasons that sent you heading for food in the first place.

You now feel great and you want to go out and socialise, rather than stay at home, feeling miserable, crying into a tub of double chocolate chip ice-cream. Maybe you are also starting to take life less seriously. Perhaps all you need to know about life can be learned from your teddy bear:

Hugs are better than chocolate
There's no such thing as too many kisses
One good cuddle can change a grumpy day
Love is supposed to wear out your fur a little
It's OK to let your inside stuffing show now and then
Listening is as important as talking
Someone's got to keep their eyes open all the time
It's never too late to have a happy childhood
Everyone needs someone to hold onto.

Anon

You may also decide that you don't *need* to lose weight.

Why do you want to lose weight?

The pressures (on women in particular) to be slim are all around us. Anyone featured in adverts for anything from chocolates to coffee, aftershave and cornflakes is slim. On television, from the woman who buys the most effective floor cleaner or uses the gentlest toilet tissue to the girlfriend who shares a piece of chewing gum, they are all slim. This is because the psychology behind advertising is that we are being sold hope, a promise of glamour as well as the actual product. It is women who respond and identify with these values - and women, far more than men, who are constantly aware of their weight and their eating habits. Whilst more men are clinically obese, there are more women who are on a diet and actively trying to lose weight. Preoccupation with food is something that women take for granted. Going on your first diet it seems is part of growing up! However, girls as young as eight have picked up their mothers' fear of food and compulsive dieting and are sensitive to the images of slimness.

There is nothing basically wrong with using slim people to advertise in this way. Any salesperson will want to put the product in its best light. A fabulous car would look crummy if it were in a shabby show room, so it is displayed with glitz and glamour to engender the dream that goes with it. Secondhand cars get the same treatment and there is even a 'new car' smell which dealers can spray into a vehicle to entice potential buyers. In the same way, clothes are displayed on slim models. This hooks into our conditioned belief that slim equals success, stunning, attractive . . . advertisers are selling a dream. The danger lies in young women (especially teenagers) internalising the image and body shape of the top models and trying to imitate them. But ask yourself, 'Why bother?' Models will always look good - that is their job. They represent the ultimate image, whether slim or curvy according to the fashions of the time. The challenge is to find ways to express yourself that make you happy and confident with your own body.

A brief history of thin

Back in the 1920's and 30's, thin was ugly. Advertisements for 'build you up foods' urged women to fill in those ugly hollows and develop graceful curves. Magazines showed women in one-piece swimsuits showing off their voluptuous figures whilst the thinnies cowered miserably at the back! A buxom silhouette remained the order of the day after the Second World War, but come the 1960's, there was a revolution. The women's movement erupted and teenage girls did not want to look like their mothers. Out went the curves and in came the Shrimp and Twiggy, with not an ounce of surplus flesh to cover their protruding bones. The new image was much sought after and, not surprisingly, the number of cases of anorexia surged as Twiggy's sparrow-thin body became the 'norm' for the fashion conscious female. A report in the *British Medical Journal* revealed that if real women were cast from the same mould as the shop window mannequins, they would be so emaciated that they wouldn't have monthly periods.

The 90's is the age of the supermodel, who is a tall, lean stick insect. Nevertheless Kate Moss took time out to put on ten pounds because she was too scrawny and looked 'unhealthy.' Now she is more like her rivals, Naomi

Campbell and Jodie Kidd, although it seems that things will be changing again soon. America is now setting the trend for the new sports models or 'UberBabes'. Gabrielle Reece is one of this new wave. She weighs more than 12 stone and is a professional volleyball player. Even her muscles have muscles but she is also a supermodel and was named by American *Elle* magazine as one of the five most beautiful women in the world. 'Strong women are sexy' proclaimed a recent issue of *Fitness* magazine (with Gabrielle on the front cover). Ten years ago her hefty physique would have excluded her from modelling; now this golden UberBabe is, allegedly, paid £22,500 for a day of fashion shoots. It seems that top models may have got as thin as it was possible to get, and things are changing. Strength and muscles are no longer regarded simply as butch, they are now feminine and sexy too.

Activate your body and mind

Taking exercise is fashionable and anyone can do it because it can mean anything from walking to rollerblading. These are aerobic activities, which are the best kind of activity to boost metabolism. They flood the brain with oxygen and endorphins, which makes you feel wonderful. The term 'aerobic' not only describes the work-outs by Jane Fonda but simply means 'with oxygen'. Any form of exercise which causes an increase in breathing and extra work by the heart and lungs to keep up with oxygen demand will tone muscles, boost the immune system and make you feel good about yourself overall. Regular exercise raises levels of endorphins, the brain's natural mood-enhancing chemicals. Laughing and having fun also promotes the release of these chemicals, so choosing a sport or activity you enjoy is a wonderful way to control stress, anxiety or depression. Anaerobic exercise (such as weight lifting) can build strength, but the oxygen factor is not there and it does not have the same all-over body effect as aerobic activity. Rather like a romantic meal, a good massage or fabulous holiday, anaerobic exercise is over too quickly.

It doesn't take long before you notice the benefits of exercise. Brisk walking uses more muscles than just about any other type of activity. You simultaneously tone your leg and thigh muscles, abdominals and buttocks. Walking works the shoulders, triceps and forearms. You can't lose - even your skin improves, making it stronger thicker and more elastic. More strenuous exercise such as jogging, hillwalking, cycling, dancing and swimming also boosts metabolic rate. This is simply the rate at which you burn Calories. Studies have found that metabolic rate is boosted by up to 19% after 90 minutes of strenuous exercise. This means that the body is burning around 200 extra Calories, over the next 12 hours, whilst you are reading, having a bath or sleeping. This effect is greater in men compared with women, but regular exercise for anyone tends to boost activity for the rest of the day.

Taking any form of regular exercise is a move in a healthy direction. Before long you'll begin to like how you feel and the confident, relaxed person you visualised will become a reality. Perhaps you feel so good that you ask yourself, 'why diet?'

Ideal Weight

When we step on the bathroom scales, what exactly are we measuring? Total body weight is made up of bones, skin, muscle, fat, intestines, organs, nerves and water. Women have an average of 35 billion adipocytes or fat cells, and teenagers do not begin to menstruate until their bodies have reached around 17% fat. In an ideal world, fat should represent 22% of a woman's total body weight. Men have 28 billion fat cells and their ideal percentage body fat is 15%. Obesity is defined as having excess body fat, which cannot be measured simply by stepping on the scales.

Are you obese?

Anyone who is fat knows that they are fat, but the Body Mass Index (BMI) is used to classify obesity. BMI is calculated by dividing a person's weight (in kilograms) by the square of their height (in metres). The desirable range for women is 20-24, and for men is 20-25. Anyone with a BMI of between 25 and 30 would be considered overweight, and above 30 obese. About half of all British adults have a BMI of more than 25 while almost 15% have an index of more than 30. The latest statistics reveal that the average women in the UK is 5ft $3^{1}/_{2}$ in tall and weighs 10st $6^{1}/_{2}$ lbs; the average man is 5ft $8^{1}/_{2}$ in and weighs 12st $5^{1}/_{2}$ lbs.

Waist size, using the humble tape measure, is another index for obesity. Women who are 80 centimetres ($31^{1}/_{2}$ inches) or less around the waist, and men who are 94 centimetres (37 inches) are safe. However, women measuring 88 centimetres ($34^1/_2$ inches) and men with a waist size of 102 centimetres (40 inches) are considered obese and should fight the flab.

For these people, losing weight means being able to tie your shoe laces without getting out of breath. Other benefits include a significant reduction in blood pressure and cholesterol levels, but the real boost comes from the tremendous psychological and social effects of not being big. Imagine you are sitting opposite a thin person on a train and they start eating a bar of chocolate. What is your reaction? Probably not a lot, as we tend to think that thin people are in control of their eating habits. Now imagine a fat person eating the same bar of chocolate. This raises much more of an issue. 'That is why they are fat . . . I wonder how many they have eaten today? . . . They have no self-control . . .' are the thoughts that run through your mind. Children as young as five describe fat people as weak, lazy, greedy, stupid, unhappy and ugly. There is no doubt that fat people carry a social stigma as well as extra pounds.

The temptation for anyone, overweight or not, is to go on a diet. The dieting industry has grown by 200% in the last 8 years, but we know that dieting is not the answer. The reason why it is so successful in financial terms is because of all the repeat business. If the dieting industry worked, we would not be overweight!

Dieting is the problem, not the solution.

8 UNCOVER THE REAL YOU!

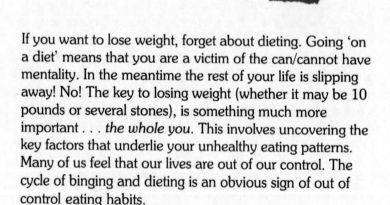

- New horizons
- Monitoring your eating habits
- Are you an emotional eater?
- Are you an external eater?
- Are you a platewatcher?

If you want to lose weight, forget about dieting. Going 'on a diet' means that you are a victim of the can/cannot have mentality. In the meantime the rest of your life is slipping away! No! The key to losing weight (whether it may be 10 pounds or several stones), is something much more important . . . *the whole you*. This involves uncovering the key factors that underlie your unhealthy eating patterns. Many of us feel that our lives are out of our control. The cycle of binging and dieting is an obvious sign of out of control eating habits.

New Horizons

A typical comment from habitual dieters is, 'You go on a diet because you don't like your body, but you end up not liking yourself!' However, there are alternatives appearing on the horizon: the antidote or anti-diet campaign, where scales are confined to the cupboard and food is not important - but you are. The anti-diet movement in America was spearheaded by Susan 'Stop The Insanity' Powter. A similar, but less raucous, campaign called 'Diet Breakers' has been set up in the UK by Mary Evans Young. The underlying principle is that 'You Count, Calories Don't.' The programme was designed by a registered dietician but rather than focusing on food, it aims to encourage people to examine the feelings that cause them to eat too much. At the more extreme end of the spectrum, this is also the approach which is used to treat individuals with eating disorders. Some of the most successful therapists don't talk about food to anorexics or bulimics - they are sick of hearing about it! Instead they are taught and encouraged to uncover the reasons and emotions behind their eating problems, before introducing a sensible eating pattern.

Monitoring Your Eating Habits

Ask any diet-conscious woman what they 'normally' eat in a day and they will run through a pattern that could be straight out of a healthy eating manual. They seem perfect and swear that they 'never eat . . . sweets, snacks, chocolate . . . or between meals.' We are very good at deluding ourselves about our eating habits, conveniently forgetting the biscuits we have with every cup of tea, or the snacks eaten in front of the television. Keeping a strict record of what you *do* eat can be very revealing. Most of us are shocked when we see a whole day's intake written

Food Diary

Day of the week _____   Date _____

Time	Food/drink eaten	Amount/ quantity	Where were you? Who were you with?	What you were doing? just before eating?	What you were doing just before eating?	Mood
7:00am	Cornflakes Semi-skimmed milk	Medium bowl ½ pint	On my own in flat	Listening to news on radio	Woke up, dressing	Happy
11:00am	Chocolate Herbal tea	1 Mars 1 cup	At work on my own at desk	Reading and typing	Really mad with Terry, my boss	So angry, feeling 'got at'
6:00pm	Stir-fry vegetable & brown rice	Large bowlful	On my own in flat	Watching TV	Enjoying cooking	Tired but fine
8.30pm	Chocolate biscuits Hot drink	5 1 mug	On my own in flat	Watching TV	Watching TV	Tired and bored
9.00pm	Bowl of cereal and milk	1 large	On my own in flat	Watching TV	Watching TV	Bored and fed-up

Food Diary

Day of the week _____   Date _____

Time	Food/drink	Amount/	Where were you?	What you were doing?	What you were doing	Mood

down for the first time. Monitoring what you eat together with the circumstances in which you ate the food, can be a very powerful tool. It enables you to identify why you eat certain foods at certain times, and can help you plan the changes you feel are necessary.

There are several ways of keeping a food diary. A good way is to buy a notebook specifically to record what you eat. Start a new page, divided into columns, for each day. A sample page with headings is given on page 112.

Aim to keep your food diary for a week or two - and be honest! In many cases the simple process of having to write down what you have eaten is enough to alter your normal pattern. Perhaps more importantly, you begin to establish a discipline in your eating habits. It may not be a very fashionable word (and it is *not* the same as denying yourself certain foods) but if you are to re-shape your life - and your body - self discipline is your means of control. Once you have a record of what you eat and the circumstances that occurred along with it, you can identify certain patterns and characteristics of your current eating habits - and set about changing them.

Are You An Emotional Eater?

The truth is that everyone is an emotional eater. We eat because we enjoy food, it gives us pleasure. Some women are plump, chubby or overweight because they want to be and are happy about it. They may feel that their size gets them noticed and big is how they want, and choose, to be. For anyone who wants to change their eating habits, your food diary can help to reveal any emotions (anger, frustration, boredom) that trigger eating . . . and overeating. For example, does someone at work (maybe your superior) really wind you up? You have to control your frustrations and irritability during the day, but maybe you return home and express your anger by eating - in effect 'rewarding' yourself for your 'suffering' Perhaps you use food as a reward to get you through the day? Do you say, 'Phew! What a workload . . . I'll do two hours and then I can have a jam tart and a diet Coke.' The pleasure we get from eating is short-lived, so turn things around. Make eating an event, not something you do because you can't think of anything better to do at the time. Look for other pleasures to reward or revitalise you. It is normal to feel tired in the afternoon, but don't confuse hunger with tiredness. Taking time out to relax or have a catnap can energise you far more than a KitKat! In this situation, try to distract yourself and find some other way of releasing your feelings. Take a relaxing bath, pull on a track suit and go for a brisk walk or jog, yell and scream or phone a friend . . . anything except eat.

Kick the habit

You need to re-position the pleasure you get from food. When you eat, enjoy it to the full, then move on.

This means breaking the habit of using food to soothe your emotions. The good news is that habits, as mentioned in the previous chapter, are possible to break - once you know how. A habit is simply a learned activity that is associated with another. You may have identified from your food diary that you associate boredom with eating. Imagine that these are two pieces of velcro stuck together. As long as they remain intact, you will always reach for something to nibble every time you are bored. Now you have realised this is why you are always in the kitchen, the trick is to gradually begin to separate the two. Imagine that you are prizing the velcro (and the association of eating with boredom) apart. Bit by bit you will have created a gap between the two pieces of velcro, the feeling and the need to eat to suppress it. The next step is to fill the gap with something else.

Active relaxation

Sometimes it may be difficult to identify why it is that you are upset. You may be suffering from stress arising from awkward times with relatives, or be tense and uptight because of an impossible schedule at work. The answer to these situations is active relaxation. You need to learn how to unwind, relax and recover before facing the challenges of the next day. Relaxation is a skill that must be learned so that you can recover and generate more energy for the next task or item on your agenda. Even something as simple as taking time out for five minutes, lying down with your eyes closed and breathing deeply, can be a beneficial beginning. Relaxation tapes with soothing sounds and music can help guide you through this process. Remember the frustrations of the day if you must, but then remember how they fit into the whole scheme of your life as you gently ease them into perspective. You tolerate a difficult person at work because basically you enjoy your job. You drive through impossible traffic because working in the city is worthwhile. Your children, whilst making enormous demands on your time and energy, are in fact the best in the entire world - but thank goodness that they are away doing homework and you have five minutes' peace!

Reclaim your life

It is in the nature of things that our lives seem to be too full or too empty. If your life, if you are honest, is not fulfilling, then now is the time to make changes. Perhaps life is not challenging enough for you? Does food fill in the times when a day drags and there's not enough to keep you busy or stimulated? This is a relatively easy situation to change, the hardest part is taking that first step. Look honestly at the way you live your life. What are your goals? What would you really like to do? Are you happy with your situation? What are you going to do with the rest of your life?

Henry James wrote about a man who had a nagging suspicion that something terrible was going to happen to him during his life . . . somewhere in his fifties, he figured out what that terrible thing was: the terrible thing was that absolutely *nothing* was going to happen to him. He was going through his entire life safely without adventure, without danger, without full participation. And by the time he figured that out, it was too late.

Setting goals

Thinking about and setting your goals does not have to be a serious event. The advantage of having goals is that they help to clarify your thoughts, give you a sense of direction and the *ooomph* to make changes. Goals can be long or short term, major or frivolous. They can be just for you or

Goal	What I need to do	When	Advantages	Barriers
Have more time to myself	No more baby-sitting. Set aside 'me time'. Talk to the family about my needs.	By Easter	I'll be less stressed & more relaxed. I'll be a nicer person to know.	The family will have less of my time. I may feel guilty.
Grow vegetables	Contact local council & apply for an allotment. Join evening class - organic gardening.	Next week New term	Good exercise. Meet new people. Fresh vegetables with a wonderful flavour	Risk of failure. No land available.
Get a part-time job	Buy local paper & scan situation vacant columns. Visit job centre. Talk to Sarah about a job share.	Every day Today	A new beginning. Meet new people. Learn new skills. Get out of a rut.	Less time with Max. Nothing local - may have to move, or travel a lot.

Goal	What I need to do	When	Advantages	Barriers

involve other people. They can relate specifically to your work, or your social life and personal relationships.

The chart on the previous page is designed to help you think about goals, how to achieve them and the possible consequences/barriers.

You may feel uncomfortable about setting goals because if you don't reach them, it sets you up as being a failure. Alternatively, perhaps you are worried if they are a success (what next?), or argue that you prefer to make it up as you go along. This may have been fine for you in the past, but you are reading this book because you want to make changes, take control of your eating habits and become the best you can be.

Imagine your future

One way to kick-start your goal-setting process is to see a vision of your future. If this works for you, spend time imagining what you want, or where you want to be, clearly in your mind. Another approach is to ask yourself: 'If I were to die today, what would I regret not having achieved?' Think about what makes you very angry or what really excites you. These questions can help to give you a sense of direction; the answers could be the basis of your goals - write these in the first column.

Sitting down, picking up a pen and putting words down on paper is often the hardest part. You may have avoided filling in your Life Journey Chart on page 87 or keeping a food record, using the excuses that 'it doesn't really matter to me' or 'I haven't got time.' This is *your* book and it has been written to help you spend time on yourself, to think about the real you and what is important in *your* life. Begin this now by putting yourself at the centre. Many people, especially women, tend to put the needs of others - children, partner, husband, parent - before themselves. A transformation occurs when you put yourself at the centre and realise that you have the power to create your world rather than letting circumstances or other people control you. Let your ideas flow. As they do, you may find yourself staring into space or chewing the end of your pen - but remember to write down your ideas. Doing this can create a powerful fear that someone else might stumble across this book and read about your innermost thoughts, hopes and dreams. A good reason to keep these pages blank you may argue! Ask yourself, is this a fear of someone else seeing the words . . . or a fear of *you* seeing them? Whatever the reason, there is no doubt that there is something very hard about committing goals to paper. To boost your motivation and confidence, keep repeating in your mind Susan Jeffers' fabulous phrase for dealing with your fears . . . 'I'll handle it!'

Once you have completed the first column, sit back and congratulate yourself. You have just created a very special list. One that will help you focus, and guide you towards whatever you want.

There are four kinds of people in the world . . .

> *People who watch things happen*
> *People to whom things happen*
> *People who don't know what is happening*
> *And people who make things happen.*
>
> *Anon*

Organise the steps

The next stage is to think about each goal and decide what action you need to take. In other words, if you have built castles in the air, now put some foundations under them. This will form the basis of how you organise and manage yourself so that you can turn your dreams into reality. Setting a time limit on your goals will help you focus and get each one in perspective. The column headed 'Advantages' is probably the most fun and may well make you smile as you relish the benefits of realising your goal. It is tempting to write 'more money' in the advantages column. This is fine to some extent: we all need money to pay the bills. But a more positive approach is to be clear about why you want the money. This distinguishes a boring activity which can only be justified because you are 'doing it for the money', from one which is a true passion and the extra pounds a convenient bonus.

Be prepared for the obstacles

The final column is to help you achieve your goals by highlighting any possible barriers that may prevent you from doing so. Setbacks and disappointments can be avoided if you see them coming and have a plan to deal with them. One of the most powerful barriers to a personal goal is the negativity of others. You may be full of confidence and enthusiasm and yet one discouraging remark can knock you flat. No doubt if you announce that you are going off around the world in search of adventure, your family might respond with cries of 'You must be mad!' or 'At *your* age?' or 'What about us?' Some of your friends might accuse you of escaping from reality . . . but what is reality? You need to find your own reality. One woman who married, moved to New Zealand and then was promptly divorced, found herself back in England with a good job and social life but still questioning, 'Is this *it*?' She used food to try to fill up the gaps in her life and was always on a diet. By chance, she went to a lecture about the work of a charity in Nepal and was hooked. She gave up her job, joined with the charity and went to Kathmandu to help build a school and clinic in a local village. Gone were the daily stresses and routine of office life. She no longer had to use curling tongs, wear make-up, or worry about doing the ironing . . . or her weight. She became a different person - calm, more tolerant and in control. She had re-discovered who she was, had lost sixteen pounds and, more importantly, her obsession with dieting.

Try to stay away from people who want to pull the rug from under you, burst your balloon or make you feel small. Seek out those who support you and want you to succeed.

Maybe you have a secret ambition - to learn to play the piano, the guitar, speak Spanish or master the art of woodwork and make your own furniture. Perhaps your fantasy is to give up your job, travel the world or meet your ideal partner? All these may be genuine enough wishes, but the challenge lies in making your dreams come true. Do you lie awake at night with a small voice inside you urging you to live for today, 'Go on, before it is too late?' The answer is to find a way to follow your dream - whatever it is! If you have any lingering fears, just remember the slogan for Nike sportswear,

. . . 'Just do it!'

Are You An External Eater?

Are you on a 'see food diet'? Do you find it hard to resist eating as soon as you see food? If there is nothing temptingly available you don't think about it, but an open packet of biscuits lying around, or the children's left-overs, are hard to resist? The answer is to practise throwing food away. This may seem terribly wasteful, but it is no more so than eating it yourself when you really don't need it. Keep tempting foods out of the house. Don't kid yourself that you need to buy cakes 'for the children' or 'in case we have visitors.'

Habit is also another trigger for eating when you don't need to. Do you associate watching videos or films with having something to nibble? If you spend all evening in front of the television this can add up to a lot of eating. The opposite habit of walking around and munching as you go has the same effect. Try to make meal times a true eating experience, sit down and enjoy having a snack, an apple or a hot meal. Keep other food away from the place where you are eating so you are not tempted to extend the meal or have another piece of cake!

Are You A Platewatcher?

A pattern that might emerge from your food diary is that you are very conscious about what you eat, and have a real fear of food. You are locked in a constant battle to control what you eat and are scared of putting on weight.

This is a very common pattern. People who ban or limit certain foods are known as 'platewatchers', and are often depressed, tired and lethargic. This is the exact opposite of 'free and easy eaters' who have a much more relaxed attitude towards what they eat. A recent study showed that a group of relaxed eaters were more energetic and no fatter compared with a group of platewatchers. They felt guilty and were locked into a vicious cycle of semi-starvation followed by binging. Do you find yourself eating more when you want to eat less? This may occur when you go out for a meal. You desperately want to be restrained, but find it difficult to say 'no'. We have all heard ourselves say things like, 'I shouldn't really.' You need to be assertive and be able to say 'no' with conviction when others all around are persuading you that it won't hurt 'just this once.' Alternatively you may be able to resist food when you are in company, but give in and lose all restraint, overeating when you are alone. This pattern of restraint followed by overeating is not easy to overcome - but you can do it. One way is to build your self-esteem (more about this in the next chapter). Stop seeing yourself as a failure. Develop your self-esteem so that it is bigger than the food which has the control over you. Change your attitude to food and allow yourself to eat . . . anything. Try to overcome the idea that enjoyable foods are forbidden and do not label things as 'good' or 'bad' foods. Give yourself permission to eat normally but keep in mind the real you - the one you want to be permanently.

Small slow changes

Having identified a link between your emotions and your pattern of eating, you can then aim to make changes - but the trick is to make them gradually. You need to learn how to relax, reduce stress, get in touch with your feelings and finally break the bond between using food to express emotions. It takes a long time to completely break an old habit - but it is the little changes on the way that are important. Pyschologists claim that it takes about 21 days to establish a new habit. The reason why many diets fail is that you are either 'on' or have broken your diet; there is no middle road. As soon as one small slip is made, all is lost and you see yourself as a failure. There are no relapses if you make gradual changes. Your goal is to enjoy and get the most out of life. If you are confident that you are heading towards this general target, then one stressful day at the office or argument with your teenage daughter causing you to slip back into your old way of eating is no big deal. The rest of this book will show you how to build your self-confidence and self-esteem, how to eat well and choose foods to improve your health. By eating foods which make you feel good, you will be able to keep sight of your target of changing your eating habits, losing weight (if you want to) and, above all, living life to the full.

9 THE SECRETS OF HEALTHY EATING

- Carbohydrates, not fats
- All calories are not the same
- How much fat do we need?
- Cooking tips
- Snacks or meals?

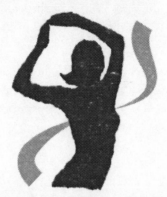

Healthy eating is all about enjoying food. It means having a healthy attitude to food, rather than seeing it as a threat. This is why previous chapters have explained how, in order to change your eating habits, you must explore your own attitude to food. If you feel guilty, or are locked into the dieting mentality where foods are classified as 'forbidden', 'good' or 'bad', then you are not ready to change.

A sensible, free-and-easy approach to food means that you can enjoy eating for the pleasure of it; nothing is out of bounds. It can be difficult for seasoned dieters, who have spent years denying themselves the so-called 'naughty but nice' foods, to cope with this free rein. But when this goes hand-in-hand with getting back in touch with yourself and your real, rather than emotional, hunger, it can be an exhilarating experience. You are free. You have broken out of the diet trap. Once you decide what you want out of life, you will see that there are far more worthwhile things to do than to be obsessed with food, thinness or your dress size. Aim to shift your goal from weight loss to being able to accept, and like, yourself - as you are *now*. With a healthy eating plan, you will not only lose weight (if you have to), but you will also feel so much better.

The secret of healthy eating is, whilst being able to eat whatever you want, to eat plenty of starchy carbohydrate foods. Exercise is also a vital part of finding and keeping to your natural weight.

Carbohydrates, Not Fats

In 1970 the average daily intake of Calories per person in the UK was 3,350. By 1981 this had fallen to 3,210 and today the average is just above the 3,000 mark. As the Bran Flakes advert would say, this is 'a step in the right direction.' We certainly need to eat fewer Calories but it isn't just the number of Calories that make up a healthy diet, but where they come from. The main nutrients that provide energy (Calories) are protein, fat, carbohydrate and alcohol. Any dieter knows that fat provides the most concentrated source of Calories and carbohydrate the least. One gram of fat will provide 9 Calories. This is over twice as much compared with one gram of carbohydrate, which provides 4. Overall, the average British diet contains too much fat. Around 40% of our total Calorie intake comes from fats and only 41% from all types of starchy and (mainly) sugary carbohydrate foods. In view of this fact, the Government, nutritionists and health professionals all agree that we need to change this fat-to-carbohydrate ratio.

The healthy eating goals mean that we need to cut our fat intake to around 30-35% of our Calories and to change the balance in favour of the starchy carbohydrates - to supply at least 50% of the total Calories each day. There is plenty of evidence from all over the world that this pattern of eating not only means that we lose weight and are able to control it - but it also means health. Once you base your eating habits on generous amounts of carbohydrate and plant foods with comparatively little protein, sugar and fat, you join the ranks of the Mediterranean people, the Chinese, Japanese or rural Africans. These are fabulously healthy people and what is more, they enjoy their food. Their cultures are based around getting together over extended meal times. They eat mounds of pasta or rice (with just a little meat or spicy tomato sauce), piles of potatoes (cooked in a tasty gravy), endless vegetables, salads and fruit with small pieces of the best and strongest cheeses - all washed down with wine or green tea!

Real food, real taste

The best thing about healthy eating is that it is not boring or repetitive. Forget the myth of having to eat nothing but lettuce leaves and lentils in order to be healthy. Overhauling yourself goes along with overhauling your eating patterns - which can open up a whole new world of exciting tastes and smells. This is eating based on real foods, with real flavour, and not cheap, over-processed

Fatty Meal/snack exchange for ...	Carbohydrates
1 fried egg, 2 small grilled sausages, small portion fried mushrooms. **Total Calories =485** **Total fat =38g**	1 poached egg 2 rashers lean, grilled bacon 2 thick slices toast a scraping of butter 2 teaspoons jam, marmalade or honey. **Calories =490** **Fat =20g**
Grilled gamon steak, grilled tomato on 2 thin slices fried bread. **Total Calories =470** **Total Fat =25g**	Large bowl of porridge with one third of a pint of semi skimmed milk, two teaspoons of honey or sugar. 1 boiled egg (cooked to perfection) with two thick slices of Marmite (no butter) wholemeal toast soldiers. **Calories =460** **Fat =12g**
1 large cheese-filled croissant. **Total Calories =525** **Total Fat =35**	1/2 French baguette filled with 2 slices lean ham, chopped iceberg lettuce, spring onions, pickled cabbage, tomato and mustard. **Calories =320** **Fat =6**
1 fast food cheeseburger with 1 milkshake. **Total Calories =650** **Total Fat =24**	2 large sandwiches filled with chicken tikka salad, 1 large banana, 1 carton fresh fruit juice. **Calories =490** **Fat =12**

Fatty Meal/snack exchange for ...	Carbohydrates
1 slice quiche garnished with salad. **Total Calories = 350** **Total Fat = 26g**	1 large baked potato, small tuna fish salad. **Calories = 285** **Fat = 12g**
Large bowl of cream of anything soup. **Total Calories = 120** **Total Fat = 8g**	Large bowl vegetable soup, crusty wholemeal roll and scraping of butter. **Calories = 130** **Fat = 4g**
2 slices of cheese on 2 slices of toast. **Total Calories = 460** **Total Fat = 32g**	½ medium tin baked beans on 2 thick slices of wholemeal toast, with scraping butter. **Calories = 410** **Fat = 9g**
1 (40g) packet of crisps. **Total Calories = 215** **Total Fat = 15g**	1 large plate of pasta shapes with small portion of spicy tomato and avocado sauce, portion of steamed broccoli. **Calories = 275** **Fat = 11g**

Table showing how eating healthily means eating more

snacks which are eaten faster than it takes to peel off the wrapper. The added bonus in eating lots of rice, potatoes, pasta, bread, cereals, pulses, peas, vegetables and fruits is that (provided that they are not smothered in butter, cheese, meat or creamy sauces) you lose weight and gain health. The trick is to avoid fat, because fat is fattening.

All Calories Are Not The Same

Not surprisingly, recent studies have shown that people who eat a lot of high fat foods become overweight and find it difficult to lose weight. Intriguingly, when those same individuals eat the same number of Calories, but in the form of carbohydrate, they lose weight. This needs some explaining!

The simple idea that we get fat if we eat more Calories than we need, is not the whole story. To return to the four potential sources of energy used by the body to provide Calories: alcohol, protein, fat and carbohydrate. In practice, fat and carbohydrate are the main fuels that are used. (Although some people do get a significant amount of their daily Calories from alcohol!) When we overeat and a high proportion of our Calories come from fat, the body - especially the female body - is very good at storing this as fat. It is an unfortunate fact that fat is stored very efficiently. There is very little (only about 4%) wastage, or energy lost, in converting fat in the food we eat, to fat stored and deposited on our hips and thighs. This is because much of the dietary fat is in the form of triglycerides which is the same arrangement as that in our adipose tissue. Triglycerides are large molecules and they are broken down by enzymes during digestion into smaller units called fatty acids and glycerol. On absorption, the body simply has to reconstruct them back into triglycerides before storing them . . . you know where. In contrast, carbohydrate in the form of starch consists of long chains of carbon and oxygen atoms - which are nothing like triglycerides. Any excess carbohydrate that we eat must first be broken down into smaller two-carbon fragments which are then built up into fatty acids. These are finally linked to glycerol to make triglycerides which can be stored as fat. A cumbersome journey, and storing carbohydrate is a wasteful process (around 25% of the potential energy in carbohydrate is wasted when it is stored as fat). It is rather like carrying buckets of water to fill up a pond. In the case of fat, only a small amount is 'spilt' on the way and it is easy to fill up the pond after only a few trips. When it is full of carbohydrate it is like carrying a bucket full of holes. Many more trips are needed to get the same amount of water (or excess Calories from carbohydrate) to its destination.

How Much Fat Do We Need?

We have to be careful not to overdo our rejection of fat and to remember that babies, children and teenagers have different nutritional needs. Not all fat is bad. We do need some to provide essential fatty acids, which are vital to health. These come from foods such as nuts, avocados, mackerel, salmon, tuna, herring and olive oil, which provide mainly unsaturated fats. Remember the aim is to keep our fat intake to a level where it provides around one third of our total Calorie intake each day. The table shows the suggested amounts of fat according to the recommended Calorie intake.

Age	Female		Male	
	Calories/day	Grams fat	Calories/day	Grams fat
Teenagers	1,845-2,110	71-82	2,220-2755	86-107
Adults (19-75)	1,810-1,940	70-75	2,100-2,550	81-99

The exact amount of fat that a person needs will depend on how active they are, their age and body weight.

The main appeal of keeping your fat intake low and eating starchy carbohydrate foods instead is that you can enjoy so much *more* food. You can relish vast quantities of starchy, high fibre foods. Whilst a high-fat snack is over in seconds, you are still munching on an alternative carbo food. It is possible to eat a whole meal for the equivalent calorific value of one packet of crisps!

The table on pages 130-31 shows how eating healthily means eating more. You will be able to appreciate these carbohydrate foods, happy in the knowledge that they will be used to give you energy, unlike fatty foods which are easily diverted to increase the size of your hips or tummy.

Healthy eating means reorganising your snacks and meals with the starchy foods (wholemeal bread, muesli and porridge, pasta, potatoes, sweetcorn, rice, peas, beans) as the basis. You may also have to rethink some of your cooking habits as well. Try stir-fried meals, steamed and dry roasted vegetables since anything fried in oil will be loaded with fat. The same is true for pasta and rice. It is the rich fatty curry or creamy sauce that can add too much fat to the overall dish.

The healthy way to eat pasta and rice is to have a large portion of spaghetti or rice with a small amount of sauce, rather than the other way around.

Cooking Tips

How To Cut The Fat And Boost The Carbohydrate

There are many ways of making recipes healthier by making them lower in fat. This usually involves substituting one ingredient for another, or changing the method of cooking. The table below gives some practical suggestions.

Ingredient/ Cooking Method	Healthier Alternative
Red Meat	Use smaller quantities of meat and replace it with beans, vegetables or pasta in made up dishes. Use lean cuts of meat or trim off any visible fat.
Poultry	Most of the fat content of chicken is just under the skin, so remove the skin before cooking and the fat comes away with it.
Fish	This is such a fabulous food. We need to eat more of it, but save the fried variety for a real treat. Tuna fish risotto, salmon stir-fry or smoked mackerel with baked potatoes make excellent meals, bursting with nutrients - and flavour!
Cheese	All hard and cream cheeses are high-fat foods. Reduce the amount of cheese in sauces and dishes by using smaller amounts of strongly flavoured cheese or adding the cheese to the top of the dish instead of in the dish. Try lower-fat cheeses such as Edam, Gouda and cottage cheese or 'lite' versions of the cream cheese. They make great sandwich or baked potato fillings mixed with chopped spring onion, watercress, pickles or chutneys.

Vegetables   Make more of these - especially organic vegetables, which have more flavour and more nutrients, justifying their higher price compared with the non-organic version.

Soups   Soften vegetables in a splash of olive oil before making soups. Use a vegetable stock or meat juices - with the fat skimmed off.

Cream   Use low-fat yogurt instead of cream or use half and half. Use this for decoration rather as a main ingredient.

Pastry   Avoid shortcrust, cheese or flaky pastry, they are all high in fat. Use filo pastry on the top of a dish only, or try a potato or an oaty crumble as an alternative topping.

Milk   Use skimmed milk or skimmed milk powder as much as possible in sauces and custards.

Sandwiches   Use less margarine or butter, or spread on one side of the bread only. Some mayonnaise-based or moist fillings do not need any spread.

Salads   Mayonnaise and salad cream contain a lot of fat. Make salad dressings with natural yogurt, herbs, spices, tomato juice, vinegar and lemon juice.

Roasting   Don't roast vegetables in a sea of fat. Chop the vegetables into large chunks (smaller pieces absorb more fat). Use a brushing of vegetable oil and bake them in an oiled baking tray.

Frying   All forms of frying will add more fat to dishes. Crinkle-cut chips will absorb more fat compared with thickly cut straight ones, which have a smaller surface area. Avoid using deep-fat frying as the main method of cooking. Go for grilling, baking, steaming or poaching.

The best thing about healthy eating is that you are not 'on a diet'. There is no need to buy special foods or cook special meals for yourself, whilst the rest of the family tucks into meat, creamy sauces and fatty fast food menus. The low-fat/high-carbohydrate, healthy eating principles (with plenty of fruits and vegetables) apply to the rest of the family too.

Snacks or meals?

How often should you eat? The answer is that it depends on you - everyone is different. Some people are morning people and don't feel right until they have had something substantial first thing. They can happily tuck into a cooked breakfast of poached egg, crispy bacon and a thick slice of wholemeal toast with jam. Others simply cannot face food at that time, and prefer to start their eating day with a wholemeal scone or salad roll at 11.00 am. What is important is that you eat for the right reasons, and thoroughly enjoy what you are eating. Make meal and snack times positive events rather than something to fill in a boring day. It takes a bit of organisation if you lead a hectic life, when it is all too easy to fall into the trap of believing that you 'can't stop' to eat, and just plough on through your work. This is fatal. Firstly you will be tempted to grab just anything to shovel into your body whilst your mind deals with a million other things, then at the end of the day, you will feel drained, tired and hungry. Again this is a dangerous time - you just want to reach for something quick and easy . . . and probably high in fat. A hunk of cheese, a handful of biscuits and a mug of hot chocolate

'will do' but these are not the best foods to tuck away.
Even busy people can make a large pot of vegetable-based
soup, or try one of the new chilled fresh soups in cartons
(avoid any tinned 'cream of' or packet soups). With a
thick slice of fresh, crusty wholemeal bread, this makes the
perfect (and fast) evening meal. Here are some other
suggestions for quick, low-fat snacks suitable for any time
of the day.

Low-fat snacks

- Marmite Muffin. Spread a scraping of butter (or low-fat spread)
  and Marmite on a toasted muffin or crumpet.

- Wholemeal bap filled with mashed banana, honey and a few
  chopped walnuts.

- Hot cross bun or toasted tea cake topped with slices of banana.

- 1 peach and a handful of grapes.

- Half a melon and as many strawberries as you can eat.

- Individual (50 gram) packet of ready-to-eat dried fruit - apricots,
  prunes, dates or figs.

- Baked apple filled with raisins and toasted flaked almonds and
  served with a heaped teaspoon of Greek or plain yogurt.

- Bowl of mixed breakfast cereals - Bran Flakes, Rice Crispies,
  Corn Flakes and Shreddies with semi-skimmed or skimmed
  milk and any chopped fruit in season.

- Large bowl of fresh, frozen or tinned (in fruit juice) fruit mixed
  with natural yogurt and honey.

- Slice of malt loaf and a banana.

Mini meals

- Greek Island snack pot. Buy a bag of ready sprouted mixed beans (or sprout your own) and add crumbled Feta cheese, chopped walnuts, toasted sunflower seeds, green olives, red pepper and cucumber.

- Mini pitta bread pocket stuffed with lean ham, lettuce, avocado and a teaspoon of tomato chutney.

- Barbecued baked beans on wholemeal toast.

- Large bowl of porridge with a handful of raisins or chopped banana added while the oats are cooking.

- Peanut butter on a wholemeal bap and sprinkled with toasted sesame seeds.

- Ham, watercress, tomato and mustard baguette.

- Red pepper and mushroom deep pan pizza (go easy on the cheese).

- Baked potato with sweetcorn, green pepper and mushroom sauce filling.

- Kidney bean, courgette and chickpea chunky soup.

- Herby baked fish with oven chips and steamed broccoli.

- Stir-fry chicken/turkey garlic risotto (use 2 teaspoons olive oil).

- Baked beans with bubble and squeak.

- Tuna pasta with Greek tomato salad and chopped parsley.

10 STEPS TO SUCCESS

- Starting steps
- You have ther power

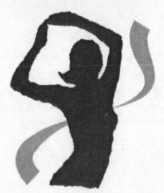

'I was always on the go and never ate sitting down. I continually munched on fast foods and whatever happened to be around. After a fried egg and bacon sandwich, hurriedly prepared and eaten on the run, I knew I just couldn't keep living like this, things had to change.'

This was a comment from a busy sales manager, who after eating her third take-away burger at 11.00am admitted that she had a problem. She got professional help and discovered that she was eating around 8,000 Calories a day!

Despite all the advice, many of us still eat badly. We blame it on our jobs, a hectic pace of living or the endless adverts for new, exciting fatty foods.

So here is a health warning: you can change the way eat.

The most effective way to change is to take a long, hard look at the way you live your life. Then decide to make some small simple changes to your lifestyle including your eating and exercise habits. The rewards are wonderful and they are waiting to be claimed.

Starting steps

Just as a journey of a thousand miles starts with a single step, here are the first steps to overhauling your eating patterns.

1 Write down everything you eat and how you feel at the time. Keep a food diary for a few weeks and examine the patterns that emerge. You will be able to see a connection between what you eat, your lifestyle and your emotional state.

2 Understand why you are eating - look at your hunger. Do you eat because you are bored, lonely or upset or do you use food as a comfort or a reward? If food doesn't seem to fill you up, then food may not be what you really want.

3 Get back to real hunger. Find other ways to satisfy your emotions. If you eat because you are stressed, then build relaxation into your daily routine. Book a regular massage or reflexology session, listen to soothing music or enjoy a catnap.

4 Change the way you think about yourself. Your brain is a powerful tool. Use positive thoughts and affirmations to boost your self-esteem and guide the way you think and behave.

5 Generate your own feelgood factor. Taking regular exercise has tremendous physical and psychological benefits. The obvious ones are improved circulation, glowing skin, protection against breast cancer, osteoporosis and heart disease. It also helps burn Calories, controls body fat . . . and makes you feel good. Any type of aerobic exercise results in the production of endorphins - the body's own 'feel good' hormones. If you are very overweight, it is best to start with a walking or swimming programme first because it is vital to strengthen your muscles and begin gradually. You can start by walking for 10 minutes a day, and increase this until you can walk briskly for half an hour a day at least four days per week. Then you'll be ready for gentle running - or anything else that takes your fancy. The important thing about exercise is that it must be something you enjoy, and be part of a regular routine. Look at the faces of those who have just been for a gentle jog or have surprised themselves that 45 minutes of an aerobics class could go so quickly. They feel great! Not only because of the endorphins, but because they have done something that they *never* thought they would do. The hardest part about taking exercise is taking that first step - past your front door! Magazines are full of stories of women who hated games at school and never thought of themselves as sporty or athletic. Nevertheless, they saw others like themselves out walking, jogging, cycling or checking into the local leisure centre, and they began to think 'why not *me?*' The great thing is that there are organisations, such as the Reebok Running Sisters

Network (see Appendix) which welcome women who feel self-conscious about starting to exercise. 'I could barely run down the road when I first joined, but now I've completed my first 6 mile race' is a typical comment from a member of the Running Sisters. Doing something you never thought you could do gives a tremendous boost to your self-esteem. No exercise programme can substitute for poor eating habits, but because you feel better, you look better and it gives you the encouragement to eat better.

6 Study your eating habits and decide what you need to change. Maybe you already eat healthily and it is just the quantity, the portion size, of food you need to change. Perhaps it is the type of food, and you need to eat less fat and more fruits and vegetables.

7 Believe that your tastes will change. How many of us buy semi-skimmed milk or have given up taking sugar in tea or coffee? Imagine going back to your old habits and you'll cringe at the thought of milk which seems too rich or tea which is too sickly. It is possible to retrain yourself to prefer lower-fat foods.

8 Small changes bring big results. Accept that you are making permanent changes. Most diets are geared towards temporary change. We want to get slimmer for summer or to fit into that little black dress. After that, it is back to our old ways. Once you learn not to diet, but simply to change the way you live, eat and cook, you have taken an important and permanent step. You will know if you have lost weight - without stepping near any scales. You will feel fantastic, your clothes will fit so well, your skin and muscle tone will improve and above all, you will feel good about yourself.

9 Have fun and enjoy life. It is important to build pleasure into a meal. Be experimental and have some fun! If your eating habits have been way out of line, or years of dieting mean that you just don't know how to eat normally any more, then you might like to set some definite goals and tackle them one at a time. Remember that journey of a thousand miles? Maybe the step you should take to change your eating habits begins with a single meal. Begin it today.

10 Stop dieting and start living. Just think, all that destructive, negative energy spent on feeling guilty and worrying about what you can and cannot eat can be turned into positive power. Who knows what we can achieve if we give up worshipping artificial perfection and start celebrating our own gifts? After all, do we really want to be loved for anything other than our true selves? Find out who you are and celebrate the wonder of your own uniqueness. You need to discover how to express yourself. Find a language that is your own and which doesn't involve food. The answers come from within. If you start to change the way you see yourself and your attitudes towards how you feel and look, you will begin to love yourself. No good longing for that mythical date in the future when things will be different.

You Have The Power

You are what you are today. Realise that you have control over your life and can do the most fantastic things for yourself and other people with all that new found positive energy. Just remember . . .

Did is a word of achievement
Won't is a word of retreat
Might is a word of bereavement
Can't is a word of defeat
Ought is a word of duty
Try is a word each hour
Will is a word of beauty
Can is a word of power!

Anon

You have read this book and know what to do. The next step is to set your goals, make a plan and take action. Stop wishing and start wanting. The facts are simple. You have the potential to let go of the past and make changes. It is time to take charge of your personal power and use it to stop dieting and start living.

Nutrition, exercise and attitude are the key determinants of fabulous health and well-being. These are all within our control. You have one body, one mind, one life. The choice is yours. After all, success means learning to make the right choices.

HELP LIST

- Useful addresses
- Further reading

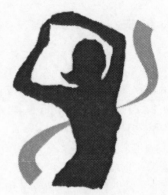

Self help, relaxation and slimming tapes/CD's

New World Cassettes

Paradise Farm
Westhall
Halesworth
Suffolk
IP19 8BR.
Send for a mail order
catalogue.

Positive thinking books from

Mindstore Direct

36 Spiers Wharf
Port Dundas
Glasgow
G4 9TB.
*Send for the latest
catalogue.*

Institute for Complementary Medicine

PO Box 194
London
SE16 1QZ.
(for a register of massage
therapists, reflexologists
etc in the UK).

Reebok Running Sisters Network (women only)

Louise Hickling
PO Box 91
Loughborough
Leicestershire
LE11 3ZZ
Send for a list of co-
ordinators in your area.

Viva! (Vegetarians International Voice for Animals)

12 Queen Square,
Brighton,
East Sussex
BN1 3FD.

Vegetarian Society (books and cookery courses)

Parkdale, Dunham Road
Altrincham
Cheshire
WA14 4OJ.

Diet Breakers (helps to build self-esteem, mainly for women)

Barford St Michael,
Banbury,
Oxon,
OX15 0UA.
Send a large sae for
details.

Eating Disorders Association

Sackville Place
44 Magdelen Street
Norwich
Norfolk
NR3 1JE
Helpline 01603-621414.

Anorexia and Bulimia Care

15 Fenhurst Gate
Aughton
Lancashire
L39 5ED
*Send an sae for
information.*

Self Development/ activity holidays

Findhorn Foundation
The Park
Findhorn Forest
Moray
IV36 0TZ
Scotland.

Centre for Natural Healing and Counselling

All Hallows House
Idol Lane
London
EC3R 5DD
Tel: 0171 2838908.

Skyros

Holidays for the mind,
body and spirit
92 Prince of Wales Road
London
NW5 3NE.

Further Reading

**The Energy Advantage:
Fuelling Your Body
And Mind For Success**
Dr Christine Fenn
(Thorsons 1997)

**Feel The Fear And Do It
Anyway**
Susan Jeffers
(Arrow 1991)

Fat Is A Feminist Issue
Susie Orbach
(Arrow 1978)

Your Best Year Yet
Jinny Ditzler
(Thorsons 1994)

Superyou
Anne Naylor
(Thorsons)

**Success Through
Positive Mental
Attitude**
Napoleon Hill & Clement
Stone
(Thorsons)

**Do It: A Guide To
Living Your Dreams**
John Roger & Peter
McWilliams

Female Rage
Mary Valentis & Anne
Devane
(Piatkus Books 1995)

Absolutely Now!
Lynne Franks
(Century Books Ltd 1997)

Help Yourself To A Job
Jackie Lewis ISBN 1-86144-033-2
£7.99 147 pp

Jackie Lewis's practical guide will give you the 'think smart' job-hunting skills you need to compete in today's tough market. She tackles head-on the special problems encountered by career-changers, or those already unemployed. Her simple activities will boost your confidence and get you thinking and moving towards your job goal right away. Jackie has helped hundreds of Job Club clients find the job they wanted using this creative person-centred approach.

Make The Most Of Being A Carer
Ann Whitfield ISBN 1-86144-036-7
£7.99 150 pp Pub Feb 98

If you are caring for someone with special needs, such as age, disability or ill-health, this is the guide you can turn to. Ann Whitfield, a social worker for many years, and herself a carer, offers expert, reliable and accessible advice covering the financial, legal, emotional and practical aspects of caring. The problems of caring can be worrying, but they don't have to overwhelm you. This guide will point you to the help you need, and show what you can do to better life for yourself and the person you care for.

Subfertility: A Caring Guide For Couples
Dr Phyllis Mortimer ISBN 1-86144-025-1
£7.99 104pp

Dr Mortimer gives a thorough and easy to understand explanation of the why, when and hows of conception, arming couples with the information they need to start looking at possible causes and solutions. She provides expert advice, encouragement and practical help to couples experiencing both major and minor fertility problems.

A Parent's Guide To Drugs
Judy Mackie ISBN 1-86144-028-6
£7.99 103 pp

Judy Mackie's no-nonsense guide addresses the questions about drugs that concern parents most, and arms them with the information they need to communicate effectively with their children. Whether you suspect your child, or their friends, may be taking drugs, or are simply worried by the horror stories and headlines - this practical guide will take you through the facts and basic steps, which you can use and develop to suit your own circumstances.

Education Matters
David Abbott ISBN 1-86144-029-4
£7.99 123 pp

Help yourself to some parent power and help your child get the most out of education. If you've ever felt confused by the new curriculum, or by school administration, don't be. Teacher David Abbott cuts through the jargon with straight facts and clear advice. Covers all you need to know, from what the Education Act means for your child, to how to check your child's real progress and talk to their teacher. Any parent can use this practical guide to help their child become a winner.

A Parent's Guide To Dyslexia And Other Learning Difficulties
Maria Chivers ISBN 1-86144-026-X
£7.99 123 pp

Many learning difficulties, once identified, can be overcome. If your child has, or you suspect they might have, learning difficulties, this essential guide gives you the facts you need to take action. It takes you step by step through diagnosis, treatment, education, and beyond into career options. Up-to-the minute facts and practical advice from the founder of the Swindon Dyslexia Centre, herself the mother of dyslexic sons.

Starting School
Lyn Carter ISBN 1-86144-031-6
£7.99 123 pp

Gives the information and advice you need to help your child to a happy and positive primary school experience. Shows how to plan for a good start, and suggests how to deal with problems that might come up. A good start to primary school lays the foundation for a successful education for your child. This book will help you create an enjoyable experience your child can build on in the future.

The Facts About The Menopause
Elliot Philipp ISBN 1-86144-034-0
£7.99 150 pp Pub Feb 98

Elliot Philipp, a consultant gynaecologist, answers the questions women most often ask about the menopause, its symptoms and treatments. He explains what the menopause is, evaluates HRT and alternative therapies, and offers practical advice on problems which can occur at this time.

This complete guide gives women the facts they need to approach their menopausal years with confidence.

Make The Most Of Your Retirement

Mike Mogano ISBN 1-86144-037-5
£7.99 150 pp Pub Feb 98

Why shouldn't you expect your retirement to be fun? asks
Mike Mogano. Your retirement can be an expanding world
of opportunity, if you organise your finances first, and look
out for problems that can come up. Plus he offers
hundreds of ideas for ways to use your new-found
freedom. Thoughtful discussion and creative suggestions
help you make the most of the life you've been waiting for.

Need2Know

Thank you for buying one of our books. We hope you found it an enjoyable read and useful guide. Need2Know produce a wide range of informative guides for people in difficult situations. Available in all good bookshops, or alternatively direct from:

Need2Know
1-2 Wainman Road
Woodston
Peterborough
PE2 7BU
Order Hotline: 01733 390801
Fax: 01733 230751

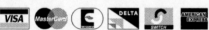

Titles